Walking Mama Home
A Caregiver's Journey

Aileen A. Gronewold

Walking Mama Home: A Caregiver's Journey
Copyright © 2024 Aileen A. Gronewold

Blue Sage Press

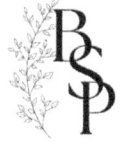

BLUE SAGE PRESS
All rights reserved.

First Edition

ISBN: 979-8-218-35591-3

Emerging Ink Solutions
Kara Wilson, Editor

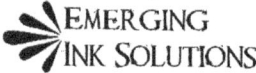

Without limiting the rights under copyright reserved above, no art of this publication may be reproduced, stored in or introduced into a retrieval system, or transmitted in any form or by any means (electronic, mechanical, photocopying, recording, or otherwise), without the prior written permission of both the copyright owner and the above publisher of this book.

Notice: This book is a memoir. It reflects the author's present recollections of experiences over time. Some events have been compressed and some dialogue has been recreated. The conversations in this book come from the author's recollections and do not represent word-for-word transcripts. The author has retold them in such a way as to elicit the feelings and meanings of what was said. In all instances, the essence of the dialogue is accurate.

To Roger
My Rock

To Elaine
My First and Favorite BFF

Introduction

IT BECAME A RITUAL. My sister Elaine and I would lie in the double bed in our parents' guest bedroom, elbowing each other and recalling epic fights from our childhood when we had been forced to share a bed at our grandparents' house. Now, here we were in our early fifties, warning each other to "stay on your own side."

"Don't make me get the masking tape to mark the line," I threatened.

"Oh yeah?" she countered. "My big toe is over the line. What are you going to do about it, Sissy?"

Eventually, the giggles and mock outrage subsided, and the room grew still. Lying in the dark, I could make out familiar shapes of artifacts from our childhood. Sameness was the very essence of coming home, the source of our comfort. In our own worlds, change demanded constant vigilance—our children leaving the nest, our careers in flux—but here, at home, predictability ruled. It anchored us to know our childhood relics would always be displayed in that same corner.

Finally, one of us said what we both were thinking.

"This may be the last time we come home to this house."

The last time. That inevitable, shadowy boogie man loomed over our every visit for several years. In our whispered conversations, we named our biggest fear The Call. Someday, one phone call would end this chapter of our story, and it really would be the last time.

Somewhere in middle age, most people face a moment when they can no longer deny their parents' failing health. More than just a cognitive nod to reality, it comes as an emotional gut punch when the implications of that decline become real. Not only will you someday lose the two longest friendships of your life, but your world will begin to intersect with theirs at a level not experienced since high school. But all the rules will be different.

Few people feel prepared.

We certainly weren't.

For six years after The Call, we walked Mama home. As her primary caregiver, I felt like I had been abducted from my own life and dumped in a foreign land without a map. I was a business professional accustomed to analyzing data, mapping strategies, leading a team, and maximizing every minute. The coming change would leave me feeling like an intern, not even sure how to make coffee.

Your choice to read this book likely means you are somewhere on that journey with a parent.

I learned, and so will you.

You may come away from this book with some practical ideas, or perhaps an "aha" moment of insight. Good. Or, just as likely, our experience may serve as a cautionary tale of what not to do. Again, good.

But this is not a how-to book. Instead, it's a "we too" book. I'm telling our story with the hope it will make you feel less alone on your own journey. Walking a parent through the final chapter of life is lonely and terrifying, even under the best circumstances. If this book enables me to walk alongside you for part of that journey, it would be my privilege.

Every situation is different. Your parents' trajectory will be different from mine. Your family dynamics, financial condition, and life situation will be unique to you. This book won't be the map you crave, but perhaps it will serve as a compass, helping to orient you in this unfamiliar territory.

As we explored this new terrain, my family discovered the four orienting points on our compass were faith, commitment, respect, and communication. With every new challenge, we relied on one of these principles to guide our decision-making.

Faith. From earliest childhood, we had been raised with a reverence for God and a deep sense of His purpose and protection in our lives. We believed that death was not the end of life, only the end of our bodies on this earth. We lived with the hope and anticipation of life eternal in God's presence.

Commitment. In keeping with our faith, we believed strongly in the duty of children to care for their parents. Mom and Dad knew with confidence that we would be there for them, to the greatest degree possible, in their old age. Importantly, my husband shared this conviction.

Respect. Not only did we love our parents, but we respected them. Growing old is one continuous series of losses—loss of health and vitality, loss of loved ones, loss of purpose, loss of control. It was especially important to us that our parents maintained agency, a say over their own lives, for as long as possible. That conviction played a crucial role in our caregiving.

Communication. The first time my parents wanted to talk to me about their will and final arrangements, I didn't want to have that conversation. But they insisted, and over time, we discussed where to find documents, who to contact for what, etc. That was the easy part. Mama and I had several key conversations as her health began to fail. Without the honesty and openness of that communication, I would have second-guessed myself to no end.

Your compass may look different from ours, but you will find yourself coming back to some core convictions to guide you. If you have siblings, it may be helpful to clarify your family's compass points with them early in the journey.

Walking Mama home was one of the hardest things I've ever done but also a precious privilege. The memories we made together forever imprinted her soul on mine. I long for the day I'll get to hug her neck again, in the sweet by-and-by, where there is no more "last time."

1
Indian Summer

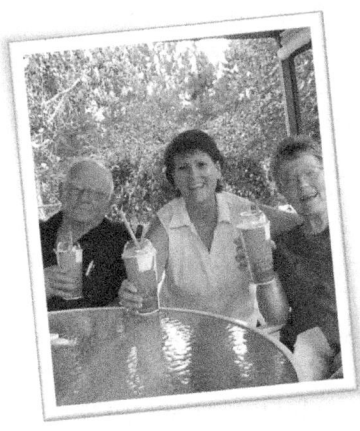

THE MOST DELICIOUS SEASON IN Colorado is undoubtedly Indian summer. Beginning in late September and lasting maybe four to six weeks, each day begins crisp, sometimes with a light frost that burns off mid-morning. Aspens, still in their golden splendor, contrast against a brilliant blue sky, and the sun warms the back of your neck. The day begs you to fill your lungs with sparkling air and praise the God of heaven for the joy of His creation. You know, of course, that winter looms, but today—today—you live in the glorious now.

Long before our caregiving journey, we determined to embrace the "glorious now" with our parents during their Indian summer. Being intentionally present with them during the autumn season of their lives smoothed the transition when they really needed us.

Our family was geographically dispersed. My parents lived in Colorado; my two older brothers, Steve and Andy, lived in Wyoming; and my younger sister, Elaine, lived in Indiana. My husband Roger and I lived in Missouri. The physical distance meant we each went about our separate lives and looked forward to occasional get-togethers. I called my folks once or twice a week and visited at least twice a year.

As much as my parents loved us, they weren't exactly pining to have us around. They had things to do, places to go, people to see. Hard to say whose schedule was more demanding, theirs or ours with three teenagers in sports.

My folks had an antiques business for years. Daddy specialized in tools and anything rusty; Mom loved glassware and all things fancy. I cross-stitched signs for each of their flea market booths—"Archie's Antiques" and "Norma's Collectibles." They had front-row reserved seats at the weekly auction, hit garage sales with religious fervor, and often helped their auctioneer friend with estate sales.

Between auctions, Daddy gardened and repaired small engines. Mom canned the garden produce and led women's Bible studies. An open garage door meant an open invitation, and friends often dropped in for a quick visit and a sample of whatever yumminess Mom had just pulled out of the oven.

They loved to entertain, and oh my, did they ever put on a spread! Their custom home graced a one-acre lot on a quiet rural street just off Highway 66, the road to Estes Park. Colorado summers begged for leisurely gatherings on the patio, where the view of Longs Peak morphed from sapphire to rose to violet as the sun sank and the crickets tuned up. Many a happy guest lingered into the night, too full of Daddy's mesquite-smoked ribs to move.

And then in 2008, Mom suffered a serious stroke.

By any objective standard, that should have been the end of the party, but it wasn't. To be sure, recovery took many months of grueling physical therapy, but Mama's stubborn streak proved a competitive advantage. She simply refused to give up.

Eventually, she resumed her old life, adjusting to some residual left-side deficit, primarily in her hand. She accepted help balancing the checkbook and lifting her canning kettle, but otherwise, she could drive herself and do most anything her heart desired.

For a while.

Balance problems caused several falls before she resigned herself to using a walker. Her hips had always been her Achilles heel, and even after repeated hip replacement surgeries, one hip had a nasty habit of popping out of its socket.

In the meantime, my burly father had his own problems. He walked with a shuffle, experienced muscle weakness, and developed a tremor. I came home to accompany him to an appointment with his neurologist, where we learned he had Parkinson's disease.

At that point, my parents were no longer just quaintly outdated. They had crossed the Rubicon. We'd been living large in those sparkling days of Indian summer, but the breeze had shifted and we suddenly shivered. Time for a family meeting.

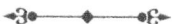

We would not be the first family to bemoan the "sandwich" dilemma—at the point your parents need you, your children are launching into adulthood, and your career hits peak demand. Each of the four siblings in our family faced constraints that made it difficult to be more present with Mom and Dad. Simple geography presented the biggest hindrance.

We gently prodded, "Isn't it time to seriously consider relocating to be in the same town with one of us?"

"But our home... our friends... our business... our doctors," came the answer.

We understood, of course, and more than anything we wanted our parents to be happy. And that meant being in charge of their own lives for as long as possible.

We siblings agreed that one of us would visit every two months, and we'd be intentional about helping with whatever needed to be done. Mom and Dad agreed to hire a housekeeper to come every two weeks and a friend to help with yard work periodically. They also agreed to keep a list of projects we could do on our visits.

Turned out that second concession was a bit soft. In casual conversation some months later, Daddy made an off-hand comment about looking at something on the roof.

"Wait, what? You climbed up on the roof?" I exclaimed.

I could picture the scene: Mom standing at the bottom of the ladder to steady it as he made his shaky ascent; the tense moment at the top when he stood up and tottered; the unsteady shuffle across the steep pitch; the backward step as he found the first rung to come back down. Even now, the mental movie makes my heart race.

My dad had always been strong and capable, and it hurt his pride to depend on others for things he had always done himself. We worked at patience and sensitivity, and he worked at acknowledging limits. Eventually, he became better at accepting help, but it was never easy.

While our every-two-months schedule didn't pan out exactly as planned, we somehow managed to make spending time with our parents a priority. As hard as it was for us to reckon with their decline, it was harder yet for them.

The biggest treat for my folks was a week each summer when my sister and I left our husbands and kids and came home to hang out with our parents. It was almost like taking a time machine back to our teen years. Once, we didn't even tell them we were coming—just showed up and rang the bell!

During these visits, we joined them in whatever activities they had planned, including water aerobics, auctions, gardening, canning, and scrapbooking. We spent a couple of days in the kitchen each time, preparing freezer meals and restocking the pantry. At the end of each busy day, we lingered over a homecooked meal and sipped root beer floats on the back patio. We all looked forward to the quiet intimacy of those weeks.

As a side benefit, we got to know and love our parents' friends. When family live far away, friends become a surrogate family. We grew particularly close to their auctioneer friend, Joe, whom we claimed as our "brother from another mother." Their tight-knit group included friends from their antiques business and church and many neighbors. We would lean on them heavily in the days ahead.

As every grandparent knows, the best way to engage a toddler is to get on the floor with him. At eye level, you experience his world from his vantage point. The same principle played out in our interactions with our parents.

By stepping into our parents' world, we learned what mattered to them. In unhurried conversations, we heard the stories of their lives and deepened our own sense of family roots. Nothing speaks love like time. Only in retrospect did we fully understand that our caregiving journey had already begun during Indian summer.

As engagement in their former activities waned, their conversation turned more frequently to bygone days. They spoke often of their childhoods, wistfully remembering "home." They each expressed a longing to go back to the old places, to recapture a childhood suddenly made precious.

It's a commonly held belief that "you can never go home again." In some sense, that's doubtlessly true, but we decided it was worth a try. The decision to take our parents home, back to their childhoods, turned out to be one of our best Indian summer decisions.

2
Country Roads

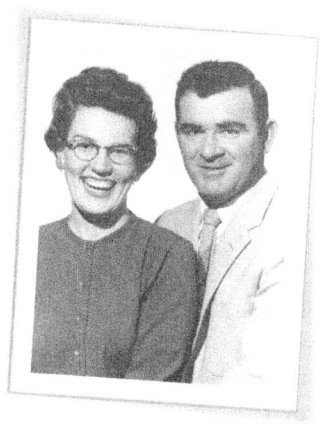

WHEN JOHN DENVER CROONED, "TAKE me home, country roads," he struck a deep human chord—the universal longing for home that most people feel at some point in their lives. Oh, how Mom and Dad longed to return to country roads from their childhoods, back to the places that had shaped them from their earliest memories.

We wondered what drove this desire. For Dad, it was partly to reconnect with his two brothers, but Mom's only sister was already gone. Most of their old friends were gone too. I suspect it was less a need to reconnect with other people and more a desire to reconnect with themselves. Perhaps, like Emily Dickinson, they might have said, "I am out with lanterns, looking for myself."

By standing once again in places they had stood as children or young adults, they returned to those earlier selves. I imagined they had questions. Had they lived up to their expectations? Had they taken the right roads? If they had known then what they knew now, would they have made different choices? And most pressing of all, had it all turned out okay in the end?

To accommodate their sudden nostalgia, we planned two road trips, one to Wyoming and one to Texas.

By that time, travel had become difficult for them. Mom needed a walker, and just getting in and out of the car required extra effort from both of them. We soon discovered which convenience stores had the best handicap restroom facilities, and we carried a change of clothes in case of accidents. Roger and I also learned to ratchet down our normal pace, walking at the painfully slow pace of octogenarians.

Wyoming

It's hard to explain the deep sense of belonging and peace that comes over me when I find myself on the Wyoming prairie with a clear line of sight to the horizon. Importantly, a jagged line of blue-violet mountains separates the prairie sage from the bright blue sky along that horizon in every direction. Many a cowboy has penned a poem or song lyric trying to capture the wonder and longing of those wide-open spaces. I totally get it.

I suspect Wesley Bloom, my great-grandfather, had the same visceral reaction in 1879 when he first reined his horse to a stop on a grassy knoll and surveyed that 360-degree vista. Wow. At age nineteen, he had come to the Wyoming territory via the Oregon Trail, wrangling rough-broke horses. He explored Montana and Idaho, hauling freight and hunting, but something had always pulled him back to Wyoming.

He had made his living as a buffalo hunter until the herds were depleted, then turned to ranching, establishing a homestead near Sheridan. In his remaining thirty years, he would also homestead in Cody and Pinedale, building successful ranches and raising a family before his life ended in a tragic accident in 1909. By the time I was born in Sheridan, some eighty years after he had filed his first homestead claim, our Wyoming roots had grown four generations deep.

Our road trip made a big loop, stopping first in Buffalo and Sheridan before crossing the Bighorn Mountains to Cody. The late September aspens still clung to the last of their gold, as if holding on just for us. We were grateful.

Mom lived all her life in Wyoming, first as a child growing up in Cody, then as an adult moving from town to town, wherever my dad's oilfield job took our family.

Thanks to the nomadic life of my childhood, we had lived in many of the small towns we passed through, and each of us had our own memories of these places. We swapped stories and stopped for photos to commemorate every stop on the trip.

In Cody, we found Mom's childhood home, or at least the place where it had once stood. We visited Heart Mountain, the Japanese internment camp from World War II, where Mom had played with her Japanese friends while her dad worked on the telephone system. We also visited Barbie, Mom's second-grade classmate with whom she had maintained a friendship for over seventy years.

I snapped a photo of Mom on the steps of Cody High School where she had graduated as valedictorian in 1954. I could picture her standing in that very spot in her cap and gown, smiling and confident. How could she have imagined that in just four short years she would marry her sweetheart, bear him two sons, and then bury him? My dad would be her second love.

In Sheridan, we saw the place where my parents met and had their first dance. She had been a widow with two little boys, living with her parents. Her dad had twisted her arm to get her to go to the dance at the Eagles Club. My dad had been working on a drilling crew in the area and had gone to the dance with some of his buddies. Reliving the first moment he laid eyes on her across the room, he shook his head at the wonder of the memory.

"She sure was a looker," he recalled.

Again, I pictured my parents at that moment. Young, attractive, full of life. Dancing. Falling in love. In the years ahead, that love would be tested. Life was just plain *hard*. What were they thinking, standing again in that same spot where fate had brought them together?

Suddenly, I thought of the Hamm's Beer box tucked away under my stairwell. Sturdy boxes had played an outsize role in our family history, and this one had met the gold standard of sturdiness. It was among the boxes they scavenged in Anchorage, Alaska in

1960 when they had packed for the first move of their new marriage, back to the Lower 48, back to Wyoming. Throughout my childhood, that Hamm's Beer box had protected our fragile Christmas ornaments through dozens of moves. Now it was mine, still holding up, still protecting the next generation of Christmas ornaments.

Standing in front of the Eagles Club again that day, I'm sure Mom and Dad weren't thinking of the Hamm's Beer box, but I'm certain they replayed scenes from their life together. Had it all been worth it? Had the spark they lit so many years ago been enough? Like that heirloom box, their love had held.

After the trip, I memorialized our adventure in a photo book. Mom savored the memories of that homecoming trip for the rest of her years.

Texas

The most remarkable thing about the place Daddy called "home" was how little it changed. To this day, the cluster of small farming communities—Weimar, Dubina, Ammansville, Schulenburg—halfway between Houston and San Antonio still feels suspended in time. Every five miles, a church spire towers above the trees next to a dance hall and the remains of a cotton gin.

It's a land where wild vines wend relentlessly up trees and fence posts, soon to hang heavy with Mustang grapes. Where cattle slowly dodge mesquite and cactus, tails swishing, to find shade beneath the low branches of a live oak. Where every house has a front porch, and the screen door has slammed behind four generations. Where the tea is sweet and the language slow.

Next to each church, those who once tilled the land and raised the church spire toward heaven, find their final resting place. The last names on the headstones—Hromadka, Janecka, Janda, Sekerka, Bartos, Mazoch, Vacek, Cernoch—tell the story of an Eastern European exodus to a promised land. Side by side, Czechs, Bohemians, Moravians, Austrians, and Germans rest from their labors in the ultimate melting pot.

This was the only world my dad had known until he shipped out for Korea at the age of eighteen.

In this community, my dad was an anomaly. Unlike his younger brothers, Harvey and Doug, he had left as a young man and never moved back. The church cemetery bears witness to the fact that many, if not most, families lived and died within a fifty-mile radius for generations. Although his livelihood took him afar, Daddy's heart belonged there among the live oaks every bit as much as his extended family.

The highlight of our trip was an evening of laughter in my uncle's Civil War-era farmhouse in Weimar. Elaine and I listened for hours as the three brothers swapped stories of their childhood.

Theirs was an ethnically-mixed family, with a German mother and a Czech father, which hardly mattered except on Fridays. That was the day reserved for religious training classes, which were held in the mother tongue, either German or Czech. Since the boys were both, they had never known which class to attend so they alternated. Somehow either choice had left them open to ribbing from their classmates.

Soon the conversation turned to their father, Lawrence, as the brothers remembered that he, too, had never felt like he belonged anywhere. Outwardly, he was as Czech as a kolache, but everyone knew he had been adopted. Who was he really? No one knew. He'd been dead for fifty years, but he had died without knowing anything about his birth family.

The mystery still bothered the brothers. Over the years, they had attempted to get information about their dad's birth family with no luck. That night they pieced together scraps of knowledge they recalled from the few times it had ever been discussed in their family. Lawrence had come to Texas from New York as a child on what was known as an "orphan train," and he had been adopted (not legally) by the Bartosh family. They believed his birthdate was May 25, 1902. That was all. It wasn't much to go on.

Elaine and I had long been captivated by the family mystery, and after that night, my sister went into full detective mode. She chased leads, poured through public records, and fought state adoption laws for months, keeping me apprised of every new clue. At last, she had strung together enough clues to know that we might find the answer at the New York Historical Society.

"Book your ticket. We're going to New York," I told her. And we did.

As we wound our way through Central Park toward the New York Historical Society, couples in bridal attire were everywhere. Having no idea what was typical for a fine autumn day in Central Park, we assumed weddings in the park must be the norm. Then it dawned on us. The date was November 11, 2011—or, 11/11/11. These couples had deemed it a particularly auspicious day to tie the knot, and as a bonus, perhaps the grooms would have an easier time remembering their anniversaries in years to come. We, too, took the unusual date as a good sign.

Finally, we found ourselves in the hushed archives of the New York Historical Society, carefully turning the yellowed pages of a leather volume with cotton-gloved hands. And there it was: our grandfather's birth certificate and admission entry in the records for the New York Foundling. Lawrence Martin, born to Delia Martin and Michael Waldron, unwed, had been surrendered to the Sisters of Charity at the New York Foundling at birth in 1902. I'm pretty sure we yelled, which wasn't allowed.

We could not wait to call our father with the biggest discovery of all: "Daddy, you're Irish! Lawrence was one hundred-percent Irish!"

At the age of eighty-one, our father finally knew his ethnic heritage. He was delighted, of course, but his identity after all these years was still firmly Czech. Finding out he was Irish was good for a laugh, but what really mattered to him was knowing the more complete picture of his father's origin story.

As we continued to piece the story together, we learned that Delia Martin and Michael Waldron had been poor Irish immigrants, barely getting by. When Delia had found herself pregnant, there was no way she could keep her job as a domestic servant and care for an infant. Her only family support had been an older sister who lived in Boston, also a domestic servant.

The New York Foundling existed for desperate mothers like Delia. She lived in the maternity ward for the last few months of her pregnancy, then surrendered her infant son to the nuns right after birth. Lawrence grew up with hundreds of other babies, the nuns his only family, until age four.

The Sisters of Charity worked with parish priests across the country to find homes for these abandoned children. Children were matched to families in advance and then transported by ship and train to their new families. When Lawrence got off the train in Weimar, Texas, at the age of four, he was being wrenched from the only family he had ever known. That day he went home with the Mazochs, a Czech family who needed a farm hand. The Mazochs likely spoke little, if any, English.

It was a bad situation from the beginning. Eventually, a lay leader in the local parish, Joseph Bartosh, staged an intervention and brought Lawrence into his family. Lawrence took the Bartosh name and grew into a quiet, industrious man. No one would ever know the pain he had buried deep in his heart, not even his three sons.

Now, at last, the secret was out. I could see my dad replaying memories in his mind as he processed this new information. How many times had he walked by the Weimar train depot during his childhood, never imagining the significance it held to his story? Now he could imagine his father standing on that platform, a frightened four-year-old unmoored from the only security he had ever known. It was nearly more than he could bear.

Growing up, perhaps he had wondered why Lawrence had been an emotionally distant father, sometimes harsh with him. Now his eyes welled with tears when he finally knew and understood his father's story. Whatever childhood wounds he may have carried found grace that day.

As I watched my dad mentally putting puzzle pieces together to understand his father, I was doing the same thing with him. Daddy was a strong man, but he had an uncommonly tender heart, especially toward children. Had he somehow internalized his father's unspoken pain? It was like looking into an infinity mirror. Here we were, seeing layers of generational trauma for the first time.

What if we had not taken that road trip, had not spent that evening reminiscing over childhood stories, had not done the research to solve the family mystery? We would have missed an opportunity to find healing and peace. Of course, we hadn't known all of that at the time. We had only known our dad had wanted to go home, one last time.

At the end of life, humans crave closure and meaning and resolution. We took our parents down the country roads of their childhoods in search of themselves. Those trips changed us all.

3
The Call

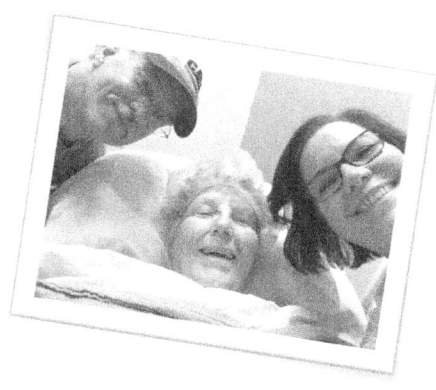

THE MORNING OF FRIDAY, JULY 31, 2015, found me in a conference room with my team of eleven talent management professionals. Our global manufacturing company had just released its quarterly earnings report, and our executives were on a call fielding questions from Wall Street analysts. We had made it a practice to have breakfast together while we listened to these quarterly investor calls.

We had a lot to cover in our team meeting afterward. Two of us had recently returned from a trip to one of our manufacturing facilities in Croatia and were eager to share our experience. With vacations winding down, we were catching our collective breath and gearing up to pitch our Vision 2020 strategic plan to our executive team. Excitement ran high.

Near the end of the conference call, I heard my name being paged on the loudspeaker, indicating I had a call waiting. Whoever was on the line had refused voicemail and requested the page, so it must have been important. I excused myself and returned to my office to take the call. When I heard my sister-in-law's voice, I knew immediately this was The Call.

Pam and my brother, Andy, were on the road, headed to Colorado. Daddy had suffered a stroke late the previous night, Pam said, and was unconscious in the hospital. Mom had called them that morning. Since Mom was waiting to talk to the doctor, they had volunteered to pass the news to the rest of the family.

An hour later, my husband and I were on our way, watching familiar Kansas mile markers tick away at a maddeningly slow pace. A phone call with Mom filled in missing details. They had gone to dinner at Aunt Alice's, one of their favorite diners, the evening before. As Daddy was getting ready for bed later that night, he had collapsed in the shower. I can only imagine the chaos that had followed.

I had tried to call my parents that very night while they were out to dinner just to see how their week was going. When I didn't get an answer, I had thought, *Oh well, I'll just call them tomorrow.*

When we arrived at the hospital, we found Daddy's condition as grave as we feared. His chest rose and fell to the whirring and beeping of machines, but he would never again regain consciousness. Still, Elaine and I held his hand and talked to him throughout the night.

"Is it possible he can hear us?" we asked the nurse.

"It's possible," she said. "We know of people who have come out of a comatose state and reported hearing conversations in the room. Medical knowledge has its limitations, so we really don't know."

We suspected she was telling a little white lie, but we loved her for it. And so, we talked through the night.

We thanked Daddy for not making us put the worms on the hook when he took us fishing. Told him how much we appreciated the example he had set to always work hard and be honest. We confessed how many times we plotted to cut down the cherry tree in the back yard so we wouldn't have to pick all bazillion of those dang cherries. We told him we simply could not face a life without his barbecued ribs, nor could we ever enjoy a root beer float again without him. He would simply have to make other plans.

The next day, surrounded by her family and several dear friends, Mom gave the okay to shut down the machines. We held hands and prayed as we delivered him into God's embrace.

For many families, panic competes with grief after the death of a parent. "What do we do now?" "Where is that life insurance policy?" "Who do we contact about his pension?" But my parents were planners. Years before, they had buttoned up all the estate planning questions, introduced us to their lawyer and financial advisor, and showed us where to find all their important documents.

Of course, as the chief record keeper of the family, Mom knew all this information. We simply played a supporting role for those times when she was too overwhelmed to process all the decisions. Still, it was heavy.

The urgent question, not addressed by their careful pre-planning, was what Mom would do now. Honestly, we all thought she would be the first to pass. Given the physical limitations resulting from her stroke, could she live alone? How would she manage caring for a 3,800-square-foot home and enormous yard? She had given up driving. How would she get to the grocery store, to church, and to doctor appointments? Most importantly, what did she *want* to do?

We siblings batted these questions back and forth while writing the obituary, visiting with friends, planning the service, and receiving flowers and fruit trays and roast beef and more flowers.

Mom's answer remained the same. This was home. Her friends… her church… her doctors. It would break her heart to move away.

We had misgivings but few options. It was all too much. Give it time, we decided. If Mom could not manage her life with the help of friends and service providers, well, she would come to that decision in time. Just in case, we siblings took this rare opportunity while we were all together to visit several assisted-living facilities. The four of us briefed Mom on our findings and chose the one we thought would be best. We left a deposit to hold a room for her and agreed to revisit the question soon.

By Friday of that emotional week, we had laid Daddy to rest and weathered each goodbye, waving each guest out of sight down the lane. It was just Mom and me for a few more days. I would help her clean up and settle a few remaining details, and then I'd head home.

Late that morning, I heard a thud and the rattle of dishes, followed by my mother's fearful cry from the other end of the house. I ran to the kitchen to find her on the floor. She was in agonizing pain but still coherent enough to say, "I've dislocated my hip. Call the ambulance."

My hands shook as I dialed 9-1-1, and after the call, I remember literally running in circles. I didn't want to leave Mom's side, but I thought I should go to the end of the driveway to flag down the ambulance. What to do? What to do? Run around in circles, apparently.

Mom was moaning in pain, and I tried to make her more comfortable on the floor. "Do you want a pillow for your head? Should I help you straighten up or change positions to take the pressure off?"

Within a few minutes, four paramedics had squeezed into the kitchen with their gurney. While three of them crowded around Mom to take her vitals and assess the situation, the one with the clipboard turned to me.

If our lives had been a made-for-TV movie, this would have been the moment when the music turned somber and the camera moved from wide-angle to a close-up of my face. In slow motion. The supporting actor had suddenly been thrown into a leading role without the script.

"What medications is she taking?" he asked.

"I don't know. I know she has several prescriptions, but I don't have any idea what they are. I'm just visiting."

Long pause.

Apparently, "I don't know" was not an acceptable answer. Try again.

Suddenly, I remembered she kept her pill basket in the pantry. Proudly, I retrieved it.

"Which hospital do you want to use?" he continued.

"I don't know. I'm just visiting," I weakly repeated.

"Can you find her ID? We'll need her information at the hospital."

"Yes, I'll get her purse." Finally, I knew one thing.

Eventually, we arrived at the local hospital ER, and the questions began again. I was expected to know Mom's every medical condition and date of diagnosis, the date of every surgery, every drug allergy, and the complete medical histories of my great-aunts.

In the exam room, the doctor tentatively moved around the bed, inquiring again about the history of Mom's hip troubles while he pressed her leg and made "mm-hmm" noises.

She had undergone hip replacement surgery on that hip several years ago, I told him. Since then, she had dislocated it several times. A second surgery a few years ago was supposed to have made it impossible for the hip to dislocate again.

"Hmm." I couldn't tell how much of this information the doctor was taking in. He was clearly strategizing how he was going to maneuver the hip back into the socket. He called in an intern and began discussing the plan.

"Wait," I practically shouted. "I think this is not your run-of-the-mill hip dislocation." We needed to get her records and maybe talk to the surgeon who fixed it last time. His name was Dr. Chiang, I told him, and she had the surgery done at Good Samaritan Hospital in nearby Lafayette.

The ER doc seemed visibly relieved. After no small effort, Dr. Chiang was located and a new plan was hatched. We would transfer her to Good Samaritan where Dr. Chiang would treat her.

Back to the ambulance, back to another ER intake process, back to the same questions again. At least I was getting better at the answers. And then we waited. I had plenty of time to bring my siblings up to speed on the latest developments.

My husband, my sister, and my brother-in-law had left that morning for Missouri and Indiana, traveling together until their roads diverged in Salina, Kansas. They had just stopped for lunch in Hays, Kansas, eight hours into the trip, when I called. My brothers had both made it home to Wyoming, eager to be back at work the next day.

My siblings' collective response to the news could be summarized as, "Hoo boy. What to do now?"

Elaine was a school teacher, and she had already missed her in-service training days prior to the start of the new school year. It would be disastrous to miss the first days of the year. My husband, Roger, was retired. Since he had no pressing obligations waiting for him at home, it was decided he would turn around and come back to be with me.

The afternoon dragged by and then the evening. At 9:00 that night, Dr. Chiang became available, and they wheeled Mom back to an operating room.

For the next three hours, I alternated pacing and trying to get comfortable in the orange vinyl chairs. The smell of stale coffee lingered in the air. One by one, the other visiting families left, leaving a deep quiet, interrupted occasionally by the squishy tread of a nurse coming down the hall.

At midnight, Dr. Chiang found me alone in the waiting room. His surgical gown was soaked with sweat, and his hair was plastered to his forehead under his cap. The news was not good. He had been unable to get the hip back in the socket. She would need surgery.

Given Mom's medical history, this news carried additional gravity. She was taking Warfarin blood thinner, which meant that she needed to wait a few days to allow her blood to thicken for surgery. My mind immediately flashed back to a scene from eight years earlier, to another conversation with Dr. Chiang. He had just performed her first hip replacement surgery and had met us in her hospital room the next day to explain in medical terms why she had suffered a stroke.

"While rare, this post-surgery complication does, unfortunately, happen sometimes," he had explained.

Suddenly, the full weight of the past week hit me. Alone in the waiting room, I held my head in my hands and let the tears come. I had just lost my father, without warning or goodbye. Would I now lose my mother too? We would have two days to think through the "what if" implications.

My brother, Andy, came back for the surgery, and we snapped a selfie with Mom before they wheeled her away to the operating room. Our next conversation with Dr. Chiang proved encouraging. She had come through the surgery just fine.

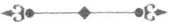

Like a slow Polaroid photo, the picture of what would come next slowly developed. But it was a blurry photo at best. Once again, everyone else went home. Mom left the hospital after a few days and settled into a skilled nursing facility for rehabilitation.

Again, I had to make a decision. The hospital social worker gave me three options for skilled nursing care and asked me which one we wanted. I knew nothing about any of them, and the social worker could not offer an opinion. No time to research, just pick one. I chose the brand-new facility, thinking she might get better care there. Not so.

The next two weeks were an absolute nightmare. I stayed with her many hours during the day but had to leave each night. If the level of care was suboptimal during the day, it was virtually nonexistent at night.

I walked past the nursing station one morning, where three nurses were deep in conversation. As I approached Mom's room, I noticed her call light was on, in clear view of the nursing station. When I went in, Mom was in tears. She had pushed her call button hours before when she needed help to go to the bathroom. No one came, and she had spent a miserable night lying in her own urine.

Need I explain the level of my anger? My immediate conversation with the director left no doubt about their negligence and the lengths to which I would go to ensure my precious Mama received the care and attention she deserved.

Mom handled it all with grace. I've never known a stronger person, but suddenly she looked frail. Life had quite literally flattened her. Each day presented a new challenge, but each day brought her closer to her release date. Finally, we loaded her into the car and headed home.

As bad as the care had been at the skilled nursing facility, I wasn't exactly a step up. I cared a lot more, but I had zero nursing skills. She needed help walking, using the restroom, bathing, and dressing. I cooked her meals, changed her wound dressing, and slept with her so I'd be close at hand if she needed anything during the night. And she did. Not since my babies were newborns had I experienced that level of sheer exhaustion.

At one point, her wound started bleeding and I couldn't get it to stop. Her blood was so thin! I panicked. I got her into the van as quickly as possible—no easy feat—and headed to the emergency room. It was the right call, and we were home again in a few hours.

While caring for Mom, I tried to keep up with my work emails and scheduled periodic calls with my team. We all like to believe we're indispensable, but the ease with which my team carried on during my unexpected leave of absence proved otherwise. I was proud of them.

I also missed them terribly. I missed the drop-by conversations, the office gossip, the funny memes. I missed outdoor lunches and game days. But as much as I missed the relationships, I also missed my work. I enjoyed the intellectual stimulation of solving problems and finding creative ways to improve a process. A few short weeks ago I was making important decisions, but none of them held life-threatening consequences.

Elaine came back for a week in mid-August. For all the unknowns, at least one thing had become clear: Mom could no longer live alone. Would she be happier in the local assisted-living facility, or did she want to move to be near one of her children? If the latter, would that be Wyoming to be near my brothers? Or Indiana to be near Elaine? Or would it be Joplin, Missouri to be near me? The choice was hers, and we assured her that any one of us would be willing to help her make the transition.

In the end, she decided to move to Joplin with me. She would hate leaving her friends and her life in Colorado, but the trauma of her injury on the heels of losing her husband had left her feeling vulnerable and uncertain. We were all surprised by her choice because she had always yearned to return to Wyoming. She would miss her mountains as much as her friends.

While the thought of having her nearby brought relief, I also felt the weight of responsibility. My job required long hours and frequent travel. How would I make time to give Mom the attention she needed? I didn't know. Like everything else in the last few weeks, I would have to figure it out.

We now turned our attention to the move. What a daunting task! I met with a realtor and signed a contract to get the house listed. Our auctioneer friend offered his services to hold an estate auction, and we set a date in September.

Back home, Roger secured an apartment for Mom at College View, an independent-living facility just two miles from our home. She could move in the first week of September, or whenever her doctor released her to travel. We knew this facility well because Roger's mom had lived there for a while too. Sadly, his mom was now in a skilled nursing facility and in the last few weeks of her life. While Roger was making all the arrangements to care for my mom, his own dear mother passed away at the end of August. It was all too much.

4
Transitions

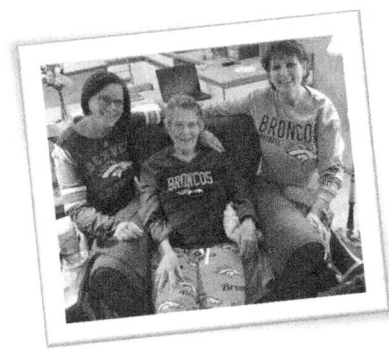

MY PARENTS HAD LIVED SIMPLY during their childrearing years, partly because we moved often and partly because money was always tight. In their retirement, however, they had embraced the joy of owning their dream home and living comfortably. Although they would never escape their frugal DNA, they managed to accumulate a lot of earthly goods, thanks in large part to being in the antiques business. Collecting was the joy of an antiques lover, and boy, did they have some joy!

Moving from a 3,800-square-foot home to an 800-square-foot apartment was going to require severe downsizing. As I walked through the house and tried to imagine it empty, I felt overwhelmed by the task.

More than the physical work involved, I cringed at the thought of the loss it would mean for Mom. Her home was an extension and reflection of herself. Every item held a memory, a part of her story. Most of the beautiful things she had lovingly curated would be sold at auction to the highest bidder. It brought me physical pain to inflict more loss on her when she had already lost so much.

I walked through each room giving myself a mental pep talk. *You can do hard things.* As if I had any other option.

Hull pottery, the passion that had first pulled my folks into antiques, could be found in literally every room of the house, including the bathrooms. We counted two hundred seventy-eight pieces, ranging from six-inch vases to thirty-six-inch ewers, each hand-painted in lovely pastels. Mom's other collections included iron trivets, depression glass, milk glass, Victorian oil lamps, whimsical tea pots, and at least eight large sets of dishes and fine china accompanied by silver and stemware and fine linens. The family room was furnished with Victorian mahogany furniture while meticulously restored walnut dressers, chests, and sleigh beds graced the bedrooms.

In contrast to her love of all things fancy, Mom had a special fondness for animals—more specifically, roosters, frogs, and moose. Each love had its own domain.

The frogs lived primarily on the patio and were interspersed throughout the gardens in the forms of decorative flowerpots or ceramic figurines peeking out among the oriental poppies. The moose had their own dedicated room, the grandkids' guest room in the basement. *No moose left behind*, I thought as I mentally inventoried the stuffed animals, figurines, night lights, lamps, pillows, and rugs.

The roosters ruled the kitchen, whose decor might best be described as Early American Chicken. Giant ceramic roosters. Hen and chicks butter dishes. Cast iron rooster trivets. Delicate egg cups with hand-painted hens. Fine china mugs with hand-painted roosters. From her easy chair, Mom directed the inventory—these to the auction, those to be packed.

When we came to the rooster cup collection, she implored, "Not my rooster cups. Please." They were a cherished reminder of the father she adored, and losing them would be like losing her daddy again. Small enough to be spared, the rooster cups went into the "pack" pile.

Eventually, we made it to the basement storage room. Aside from Christmas decorations and luggage, canned goods comprised most of this inventory. For years we had joked that if the country ever faced another Great Depression, we would all move home because Mom and Dad had stockpiled enough food to feed us all for a year! Garden bounty filled two extra freezers and numerous shelves. One weekend, we loaded my brother's pickup with boxes of home-canned beets, green beans, tomato sauce, jellies, pickles, and salsa. Thankfully, his large family made good use of everything.

Somewhere in the process, I discovered that my meticulously organized mother had never purged a piece of paper in her life. She had boxes of old bank statements, pay stubs, tax returns, and correspondence stashed in the guest room closet. We stacked the boxes in the living room, and when we were too tired to move, we'd push ourselves to get through a box or two. I'd sit on the floor and dig through the contents, setting aside anything with personal information that would have to be shredded.

Each box took us back to an earlier chapter in our shared story. Back to the Before Time, when we might expect Daddy to walk through the door at any moment, his shop apron covered in grease from whatever small engine he'd been working on. Grief that had been suspended by Mom's accident now roared back. Each day left us physically and emotionally drained.

We finally made it through every room in the house, but we hadn't touched the garage. Daddy's workshop, the size of a four-car garage, was piled high with boxes of screwdrivers, wrenches, hammers, sockets, and planes. Bins of screws, nuts, bolts, and washers. Pieces of small engines, coils of wire and rope, and extension cords in various lengths. Anvils and vices, lawn tools and snow shovels. It was Man Heaven.

As my eyes swept the shelves and workbenches for this mental inventory, I noticed the green ledger pad where he recorded his purchases and sales. The sight of his distinctive handwriting, still precise despite his Parkinson's disease, hit me with a physical pang. On the day he died, he had recorded a few purchases, then laid his pen diagonally across the pad, intending to return later to finish.

Obviously, nothing in the shop would need to be moved to Joplin, but what on earth were we going to do with all of it? We did not have the energy or imagination to address it.

By the end of August, we had a solid plan. The first week of September, Roger returned to Colorado, and we packed a U-Haul with most of Mom's belongings. Elaine and her husband, Dan, also returned. They would stay with Mom for what we hoped would be only a week, pending the doctor's release, then drive her to Joplin.

Roger and I spent Labor Day weekend unpacking Mom's belongings and setting up her new home at College View. We crashed in utter exhaustion Monday night, but it was nice to be home and to be together again. We felt like earthquake survivors digging out of the rubble, which we were, metaphorically speaking. But the calm was premature. An aftershock loomed for me.

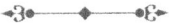

The Tuesday after Labor Day, I woke early. I'd been gone from the office for five weeks and I could not wait to reconnect with my team. I had the rare good fortune to work with a group of highly talented and downright fun colleagues. With eager anticipation, I pulled professional clothing out of my closet—a welcome change!—and got ready for work.

At 8:30, I still hadn't made it to my office because I had stopped to chat on my way. My assistant poked her head into the room and told me I had a call from my boss, Joe. I hurried to my office and cheerfully greeted him. He said he was in a conference room with James, another colleague from our Human Resources department, and they needed me to stop by. I hurried across the building to join the meeting.

It took only seconds to realize this was no ordinary meeting. Without any cursory small talk or inquiries about my mom's health, Joe launched into the "we've decided to go another direction" spiel. I was being fired. My heart thumping wildly, I tried desperately to connect dots in my head, but the dots were swimming and refused to align. How could this be? Finally, I blurted out, "But, why?"

Joe snidely offered to give me a list of my shortcomings, but I declined the offer. The dots had aligned by this time, and I knew why. Our relationship had been strained for some time, and my extended absence had given him time to put a plan in place.

Within minutes, James was escorting me back to my office. He had a stash of boxes nearby, which he carried into my office, closing the door behind him. I caught a glimpse of my assistant's shocked face before the door closed. James explained the next steps calmly while I started filling the boxes with my personal effects. As the employee relations guy, he had done this a thousand times. Still, I could tell he was deeply uncomfortable.

He informed me that my computer access had been shut off while we were in the meeting. I would receive a severance offer soon that would lay out the conditions upon which I would receive severance compensation. "Of course," he said, "you may wish to consult legal counsel before you sign it, but you will need to respond within seven days."

I asked if I could have a few minutes to say goodbye to my team. He shook his head, "No. When you're finished, we'll get a cart for the boxes, and I'll walk you out. I'll need your key card and office key. If you have any questions regarding the severance offer after you've had a chance to review it, call me."

And thus ended a seventeen-year-long career I had loved.

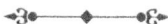

The rest of that week felt like the first few moments after stepping off a Tilt-a-Whirl at the state fair. The spinning had stopped, but it hadn't yet registered in the brain. The feet were unsure, cautiously testing the ground to see if it would hold. The stomach lurched, and everything seemed *so loud*.

I ran through a cycle of emotions several times a day—anger, embarrassment, confusion, panic, regret, sadness, outrage, shame, betrayal, paralysis, and even relief. I tried to focus on the immediate decision facing me: whether to accept the proposed severance or reject it to preserve the option of legal recourse. I sought the advice of trusted friends and crunched numbers in our financial planning spreadsheet.

Over seventeen years, I'd accumulated a wealth of meaningful relationships within the company. To be escorted out of the building without a chance to say goodbye cut me deeply, but those friendships remained steadfast. I got so many texts, Facebook messages, cards, visits, and phone calls (several from executives) that I had to start a list to keep track. On the really dark days, I read through the list.

It was months before I found my equilibrium, but by the time Mom arrived, I could at least breathe again. I leaned into my faith, knowing that God held my future and I could trust him completely.

That weekend, Dan and Elaine arrived with Mom. I'll never forget the childlike joy on her face when we ushered her into her new home. She exclaimed anew over every one of her belongings, arranged just as we knew she would like them. Her couch and recliner, her pictures on the wall, her favorite throw, her teakettle, family photos everywhere, new lavender towels in the bathroom, and her rooster cups just where they belonged in her kitchen. It felt like home, and she could not contain her joy. After weeks of packing and living in chaos, she melted into her recliner and exhaled. Of course, she still had many adjustments ahead, but in that moment, she appeared confident.

By the time Dan and Elaine headed home, we had only one remaining task on our to-do list. All four siblings would reconvene in Colorado for the estate auction the following weekend. We felt confident the house would sell quickly, and this would be the dreaded "last time" we would come home to this place of so many shared memories.

We all arrived a few days in advance of the auction to help prepare. We still had no idea how to handle sorting through the contents of the shop, but three of Daddy's close friends stepped forward and volunteered to go through everything and organize it for the sale. Sometimes angels wear greasy shop aprons and know the difference between an Allen wrench and a crescent wrench.

By that time, each of us had already taken home many keepsake items. Still, it was hard to watch things we knew were precious to our parents being set out for auction to the highest bidder. Our memories were being valued by strangers. We were thankful Mom had opted not to come for the auction, especially when the day's proceeds barely covered its expenses.

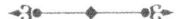

Those first few weeks following Mom's move to Joplin were filled with adjustments for both of us. On the bright side, I no longer had to wonder how I was going to fit Mom into my busy schedule. Suddenly, my calendar was wide open.

Mom soon adjusted to the dining schedule of the facility. She fixed her own breakfast but went to the dining room for lunch and supper. Tables of four had assigned seats, so she quickly came to know and like her tablemates. I had hoped she would participate in social activities or join a puzzle table, but she had no interest. She was happy in her little apartment and could always entertain herself with a book, a puzzle, or games on her iPad.

I spent time with her every day. She received housekeeping service once a week, but I helped her with her laundry, purchasing and hauling groceries, and any number of small homemaking tasks. She was always up for a day trip or an outing to Macy's or the antiques mall. And of course, we had doctor appointments at least once a month because of the need to monitor her blood thickness.

She missed my dad, and she missed her friends. She grieved those losses but remained amazingly positive. To her surprise, she found several advantages to her new independence. My dad had always favored eating at home, so Mom rarely got to enjoy her favorite Taco Bell entree. Now, she could have Taco Bell any time she wanted it, and she did! We ate Taco Bell several times a week until she finally got her fill.

I have never seen my mother's faith shaken. At a time when I should have been comforting her, she often ended up comforting me. The loss of my career hurt deeply. As I vacillated between anger and self-flagellation, she remained a steadfast sounding board. I was fifty-five years old, but it still felt so natural to go to my mama with my hurt.

The deepest cut was the betrayal I felt from my boss, a man I had once counted a friend. Mom had experienced betrayals deeper than mine, and she could empathize. She listened patiently and without judgment. When I talked about egging my former boss's mailbox, she calmly weighed the pros and cons. When I beat myself up over my mistakes, she reminded me that I was human and nothing was irredeemable.

And when my former boss got fired a few months after my sudden exit? Well, let's just say Mom did not judge me for feeling a certain gleeful vindication.

We settled into a routine, but I was anxious about the financial impact of my unemployment. I had accepted the severance agreement, and that compensation helped, but only marginally. Roger was already retired. Could I afford to retire at fifty-five? If not, what kind of position would allow me the flexibility I needed to care for Mom?

It soon became clear that my new caregiving responsibilities were incompatible with a full-time job at a similar level, even if I could find one. I did occasional consulting, tried a sales job, and did bookkeeping for my son-in-law's business. The amount of time and income involved in those side gigs, however, proved so minimal that I couldn't even consider myself "semi-retired." Eventually, I was able to relax and trust that our nest egg was sufficient. I gave up the job search and just accepted being retired sooner than planned.

After the initial shock, I enjoyed the freedom of an open calendar. I had longed for more time with my husband, children, and grandchildren, and so, I embraced every opportunity to do just that. I had also dreamed of pursing my love of writing, and I soon launched a lifestyle blog. It felt good to be devoting time to my passions.

The hallways at College View had a certain college dorm feel. Each apartment had a small shelf beside the door where residents displayed family photos or military memorabilia or indications of a favorite hobby. Walking down the hall, these decorated shelves gave a sense of the personalities and stories behind every apartment door.

Mom's shelf displayed moose, of course, but changed for every holiday and season. In fact, these shelves and the wreaths on each door reliably chronicled the rhythm of senior life. Valentine's hearts gave way to shamrocks, then to Easter bunnies and lilies, followed by American flags. Autumn brought pumpkins and mums before yielding to turkeys and Santas. Mom loved it all and delighted in the Hobby Lobby runs that preceded each change.

A great fan of essential oils, Mom took joy in using her diffuser to fill her home with her favorite scents. Unfortunately, her inability to add just a drop or two of oil meant that her scent-of-the day often filled the entire hall! Stepping off the elevator, I knew immediately when Mom was feeling peppermint.

Mobility remained a challenge, but Mom managed. Over time, I started to notice some mental confusion. She would sometimes lose herself down a memory hole and have a difficult time shaking off negative emotions. This was unusual behavior for her, and I worried that the amount of time she spent alone was proving to be detrimental to her mental health. I took her out at least once a week and spent time with her every day, but it was just a tiny fraction of the time she spent alone. I felt guilty for not spending more time with her.

In October 2016, Roger and I made a day trip to Kansas City to spend the day with our youngest daughter and celebrate Roger's birthday. Mom had been in her apartment just over a year by this time, and she was self-sufficient enough that we didn't worry about being gone for the day. A few hours into our excursion, however, a phone call from College View changed our plans. It appeared that Mom had dislocated her hip. They had found her on the floor beside her apartment door and called an ambulance.

We were two and a half hours away but turned around and got there as quickly as we could. By the time I arrived at the hospital, the hip was back in place. Whether it had fully dislocated or not, we couldn't be sure. One thing was certain: the hip could not be trusted. An orthopedic doctor fitted her with a brace that cinched around her waist and had a metal bar extending to her knee. This immobilized the leg enough, in theory, to prevent another dislocation.

I stayed with Mom at her apartment for a few days while she got used to the brace. It was cumbersome and uncomfortable, and she had to remove it to go to the bathroom. With only one functional hand, she could not manage it alone.

At a follow-up orthopedic appointment, we discussed the possibility of another surgery to better secure the hip, but the surgeon was skeptical. I had flashbacks to the five weeks I had spent in Colorado just a year before, helping Mom recover from the last hip surgery. Neither of us wanted to go through that again.

What to do? Mom now needed more help than was readily available at her apartment complex. Could we hire someone? Should we move her to an assisted-living facility? Roger and I discussed the possibility of moving her in with us.

In some ways, it would be a relief to have her live with us. It would reduce my feeling of being torn between two worlds if the worlds were merged. I wouldn't worry about her as much. In the current arrangement, I was always waiting for the next call. If she lived with us, I would be able to tell if her hip was going wonky again. I was also sure that increased human interaction would help her mental stability. Besides, I would enjoy her company.

However, we also knew we'd be giving up our privacy. Would we still feel like we could have friends over for dinner or to play cards? We would be more tied down. Could we find a way to still make short trips? I would need to have some time away. Mom had a long-term care insurance policy that would enable us to hire caregivers when we needed to be gone, but clearly, it was going to require most of my time to care for her.

Overall, we thought the pros outweighed the cons. We would figure it out, just as we had done up until that point.

After consulting my siblings, we decided this was the best option. I proposed that the money Mom had been paying for her apartment rent, be paid to us for her room and board. Whereas I could have taken a job before, now caring for Mom would be my job. My siblings agreed that redirecting her rent payments to us was an appropriate compensation for my services. We all knew the assisted-living alternative would have been much more costly.

We presented the options to Mom, and she jumped at the chance to come live with us.

We lived in a 1940s rock cottage that we had gradually expanded from 850 square feet to 2,000 square feet by adding a kitchen and finishing the basement and attic. We had added a back porch when we built the kitchen and leveled it with the driveway. What fabulous good luck that Mom would have no steps to navigate.

Although our home has five bedrooms now, our bedroom was the only one on the main floor of the house. Fortunately, we had recently renovated the main floor bathroom and replaced the tub with a walk-in shower, complete with hand rails and a hand-held shower head. It would be easy enough to settle Mom into our bedroom with effortless access to the bathroom.

Once again, we packed her belongings, scaling down her earthly goods even further. A new chapter had begun.

5
Family Ties

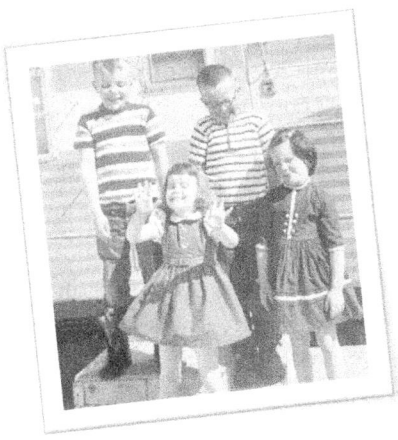

CAREGIVING DECISIONS RIGHTLY FOCUS ON the prospective caregiver and the parent. It's easy to minimize, or fail to recognize at all, the impact caregiving may have on other relationships—spouses, children, siblings, and even friends. Over time, a commitment to caregiving necessarily requires a re-ordering of priorities, which cannot help but impact relationships, at least for a time.

Before inviting Mom to move in with us, Roger and I had talked through the implications to our marriage, as far as we understood them. But honestly, we were largely jumping off a cliff into the unknown.

And that, friends—the unknown—is the biggest quandary of caregiving. All the planning and communication in the world matters naught against the great unknown. You have no idea if you are committing to six months or six years. You cannot know what degree of physical and mental decline is in the cards for your parent.

Furthermore, the world keeps turning while you are busy caregiving. What macro external forces might you face on this caregiving journey? An economic recession, political chaos, a pandemic? What disruptions might hit closer to home? A devastating diagnosis, a required relocation, a job loss, a divorce?

Roger and I held strong convictions about our duty and desire to care for our parents in their old age. In spite of that, we would not have invited Mom to move in with us had we believed our marriage to be tenuous. Our marriage took priority.

As it turns out, however, our marriage had some fault lines that only became apparent in hindsight. We entered our caregiving season with thirty-seven years of marital history and deeply ingrained patterns. As empty-nesters, our marriage had puttered along pretty well on auto-pilot. But auto-pilot doesn't cut it when a parent moves in. Even though our intentions and convictions were in sync, our relationship felt the strain as the years passed. Once committed to caregiving, however, it was difficult to change course.

Even in loving families, the burden of caregiving is never evenly distributed. Sometimes from childhood, it's clear which child will be the designated caregiver, and it's often the firstborn daughter. In our family, it could easily have been either me or my sister. Once the designated caregiver assumes that role, it's natural for everyone else to grow comfortable in supporting roles.

I wish I had said to my siblings on the front end, "Yes, I am willing to be Mom's primary caregiver. But I'm going to need your help. There may come a day when I am unable to continue in this role. Keep that in the back of your mind because you may need to come off the bench at some point in the future. We're all in this together."

I don't mean to imply that my siblings did not support me. They certainly did to the degree they could. Elaine was my most ready aide, volunteering to take Mom for several weeks in the summer and sometimes over Christmas. Eventually, however, I needed more help than that.

We had seen this play out in Roger's family. When his dad died, his older sister had gladly taken on the caregiver role for his mom, moving her to an independent-living facility near her in Arizona. But a few years later, his sister had been diagnosed with breast cancer. There was no way she could continue to care for her mother while undergoing treatment, so Roger had assumed the primary caregiver role and moved his mom to Joplin.

Does the shared responsibility for a parent's care need to be stated upfront? Maybe not, but clear communication on the front end would have made our situation easier. Roger and I were fortunate to have strong bonds of mutual love and respect with all our siblings. Not everyone has that advantage. Even so, it's challenging to pass the caregiving baton.

There were other challenges, too, long before our crisis point. For all the thoughtful consideration my siblings and I had given to our relationship with our parents, we had given zero thought to how a caregiving scenario might impact our relationships with each other.

As Mom's caregiver, I felt the responsibility to keep everyone informed. Most of my communication happened informally, one-on-one, in the course of our regular phone calls with each other. Sometimes I sent a text or email to give them all an important update on Mom's health.

Years before my dad's death, I had agreed to be the trustee of my parents' trust and to be their healthcare power of attorney. I had not considered how delicate it might be to balance that decision-making authority with the interests of my siblings. After all, they were important stakeholders too. What happened if we didn't agree on something?

It was more challenging than I might have imagined to find the right balance when we faced important health decisions. It rarely came up with my brothers, but Elaine and I often held different perspectives.

In hindsight, the potential for conflict between my sister and me made sense. Only a year apart, we had always been close. We had looked a lot alike when we were young, and people could never keep us straight. Aileen? Elaine? Are you girls twins? We heard it all the time.

Although we looked alike, our personalities were very different. She was a fun-loving extrovert; I was a reserved introvert.

Perhaps nothing illustrated our personality differences better than the Great Schulenburg Tomato War, an incident of childhood naughtiness with our cousins, the retelling of which gets better with age. Accounts differ, but I remember her being among the first to throw one of Aunt Cleo's ripe tomatoes in an epic battle that ended with seven cousins wearing a full bushel basket of cherished tomatoes. I recall being on the fringes of the action, too guilt-ridden to actually pick up a tomato. Elaine had jumped in with both feet and considered the fun worth the punishment.

Our personality differences had seemed to magnify in our teen years. She was a star athlete; I was a bookworm. She was David Cassidy; I was Donny Osmond. While she was traveling to a ball tournament, I was home sewing a new outfit.

For all our differences, she was my constant playmate in childhood and has remained my first and dearest friend throughout our adult lives. We were both very close to Mom.

The first time we faced conflicting opinions came when we were considering another hip surgery for Mom. I was deeply reluctant, but Elaine thought we should do it. As the person who would be living through the recovery, I felt my opinion carried more weight, but I also knew I would want my views to be considered if our roles had been reversed. Fortunately, Mom was able to weigh in on that decision, and we decided against it.

Later, we faced some tricky decisions at the height of the COVID pandemic. Roger and I took every precaution possible to prevent exposing Mom to the virus. We masked, avoided crowds, canceled travel plans, and got the vaccine as soon as it became available. The rest of the family took a more relaxed approach to COVID, resisting masks and vaccines.

It was easy enough to accept the differences in their precautions until family members wanted to visit. Of course, Mom longed to see them. What to do? At the time, she was fully capable of weighing in on the decision, and we came to a solution acceptable to everyone. Roger, Mom, and I accepted a higher degree of exposure risk in exchange for the family taking greater precautions before and during the visit.

Another factor I had not considered was the weight of responsibility I felt in managing Mom's finances. When my parents had designated me power of attorney for their trust, I hadn't given it much thought. But when I actually assumed that responsibility, it felt daunting. I was making decisions that affected not only Mom but each of my siblings as heirs.

To be clear, Mom and Dad's investments were managed by a trusted broker at a reputable investment firm. At first, Mom and I had both participated in the periodic calls with her broker, but it had quickly become apparent that she was not really understanding much of the conversation. As she became comfortable with me managing her finances, she opted not to participate in the calls.

Even with professional management, I understood the need for us to have proactive oversight of her investment portfolio. My parents had been through a bad experience with a broker years before, and they believed poor management had cost them serious financial loss. Even though they trusted their broker, I knew my dad had been deeply involved with the management of their investments. While I had a fair amount of financial knowledge, having full oversight responsibility felt heavy.

I talked to Mom about it and asked her to consider amending the trust document to add my brother, Andy, as a trustee. We would be co-trustees, but we each had the ability to act independently. We talked to Andy and consulted her lawyer. The lawyer cautioned us about potential problems with that arrangement, but after weighing all the factors, we thought it was the best move for us.

After that, I consulted with Andy frequently about investment decisions. His work schedule prevented him from participating in the calls with the broker, but I would send him a detailed summary afterward. It was good to have his help with other financial decisions, including the decision to increase the monthly stipend Mom paid to us for her care as the caregiving demands increased. I was grateful for his insight, and it was a safeguard for me to have a sounding board.

Even in the day-to-day management of Mom's finances, I kept records and receipts. I could not imagine my siblings ever asking for an accounting of my financial management, but I understood my fiduciary role and never wanted there to be any room for doubt.

Looking back, there were so many challenges we failed to anticipate. We figured it out as we went, and fortunately, our relationships withstood the challenges.

6
Sharing Space

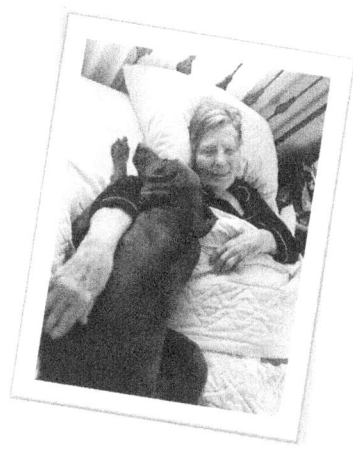

THE LAST TIME MOM AND I had lived under the same roof, I had just graduated from high school and was planning my wedding. A few things had changed in the intervening years!

Moving her in and rearranging our own belongings proved easy. We had recently purchased a memory foam mattress for our bed, and it was just perfect for Mom. Her new bedroom was smaller than the last, but everything she needed fit with just enough room for her to squeeze by with her walker.

Our vintage wrought-iron bed beautifully complimented her Victorian decor. We hung her crystal pendant light in the corner, placed the "Norma's Collectibles" cross-stitch picture from her antiques booth on the wall, and draped three of my dad's beautiful silk ties from decorative knobs. I made the bed with her favorite quilt and arranged silk roses in a delicate yellow vase on her dresser. She exclaimed with joy every time she went into the room for months. It felt like home.

Some of Mom's other favorite items found places throughout the house. We added her books and photo albums to our bookcase, found room for her favorite dishes in the kitchen, and displayed her rooster cup collection on the kitchen windowsill. To her great chagrin, I drew the line at her beloved diffuser. I was happy to enjoy a candle with her, I said, but I simply could not tolerate her essential oils. It nearly broke her heart.

For Mom, one of the best things about living with us was Rawley, our redbone coonhound. They loved each other. Rawley would jump up on Mom's bed in the morning, liberally kiss her, then settle in for a little snuggle on her pillow. Mom would shriek and giggle, and we all started the day on a happy note.

Our tiny bathroom was too small for me to be able to help her, so we put a bedside commode in her bedroom. That gave me enough room to stand on either side of her to help with the brace, and I found that, aside from the brace, she needed help anyway. She struggled with incontinence, and it became typical to change her undergarments a couple of times a day.

I lived in constant fear of her falling. I put a baby monitor on the nightstand so I would hear her when she awoke and needed to go to the bathroom, which she did at least once each night. For the first few weeks, every time she snored or sighed in her sleep, I sat straight up in bed, my heart pounding. Eventually, I got comfortable enough to turn the monitor off.

Mom's bedroom adjoined the living room, so it was only a few steps from her bedroom to her small recliner, which had an electric mechanism to raise and lower the footrest. A table beside her chair held Kleenex, her phone, and small essentials while a basket below held her books and iPad. Instead of coming to the kitchen for meals, we brought meals to her. A small lap desk made a perfect table.

Before Mom moved in, Roger and I had been very relaxed about meals. I cooked a few times a week, but cooking for two seemed like a lot of trouble, so we often foraged for whatever we could find in the fridge. And who's to say that cold cereal cannot be supper?

With Mom's sudden company, I needed to cook three meals a day. Because she was on Warfarin blood thinner, she could not eat several of our favorite foods, including salads. Mom was not a picky eater, but the things she loved most happened to be things I could not abide. Like pickled beets and fried okra. Gah. It took us awhile to settle into some mutually acceptable menus.

Mom needed help dressing and undressing, especially with the brace. She could brush her teeth but often needed a little help with her hair. She could not trim her fingernails, and we engaged outside services for foot care. She had lived with us for a full week before I found the gumption to tackle the biggest learning curve: showers.

Instead of using a shower chair, we found that her bedside commode, with the pot removed, worked just fine. The biggest challenge was getting her into the shower in such a small space. She had great difficulty lifting her left foot, and the shower had a three-inch lip that sometimes took several minutes to navigate.

When we remodeled the bathroom a few years earlier, we had done so with just this scenario in mind. We had thought the walk-in shower was a brilliant move. How could we have known that the three-inch curb would be such a problem?

And can I just admit, please, that it's a little disconcerting at first to see your parent naked? Mom had suffered so many indignities with her poor old body by this time, she had no inhibitions left. But for me, this level of intimacy with my mom took some getting used to.

Life soon established a predictable rhythm, but Roger and I felt the lack of privacy. The cozy dimensions of our house meant there was no place to speak privately. The large shop beside our house where Roger had once run his collision repair business became our best option for private conversations.

Despite these more difficult adjustments, Roger was fully on board with our decision to care for Mom and became highly solicitous of her comfort. She was almost always cold, and he happily set the thermostat at an unbearable seventy-eight degrees to accommodate her. I reminded him that I needed to be able to breathe, and we eventually found a thermostat compromise that had me wearing shorts in December and Mom bundled up in plush throws.

We also made entertainment compromises. Roger and I found a certain vintage charm in old *Lawrence Welk* and *Perry Mason* episodes while Mom gritted her teeth through episodes of *The Voice*.

Music was a great source of comfort for Mom. She loved Jim Reeves, Daniel O'Donnell, and instrumental worship music best of all. Occasionally, we indulged in classic country with Hank Williams, Patsy Cline, and Ernest Tubbs, the soundtracks of my childhood.

We spent a good part of each day just visiting. One of our projects was to go through all her photos. Mom had been an avid scrapbooker a few years earlier and had made several beautiful albums. But she still had many loose photos, as well as older albums, with no documentation to identify the people and contexts of the photos.

One afternoon, we went through a stack of senior photos of the Cody High School class of 1954. She remembered each classmate clearly and told me story after story about each one. In the normal course of our lives, we'd never had occasion to talk about the details of her experiences in high school, and I relished the chance to hear them.

We shared a common interest in our family history, and I had embarked on some serious research into her lineage, specifically my great-grandfather, Wesley Bloom. Mom had been fascinated by Wesley's life and had worked on that research periodically for years. With her typical penchant for organization, she had binders of family history information and walked me through all the pieces of the puzzle she'd been able to find. In the years to come, I would delve deeper into Wesley's life, and each discovery in this joint project sparked our mutual excitement.

As we paged through the oldest albums, memories from her early childhood bubbled to the surface. I wish now that I had recorded some of those conversations, but on the other hand, it might have killed the mood. The spontaneous tidbits that came up naturally in casual conversation helped me see my mother through a different lens.

She told me about difficulties in her relationship with her mother, something I had never known. She had only one sibling, an older sister, and in her mind at least, each parent had a favorite. Her mother had favored her sister, and her dad had favored her. The dynamic had left some scars on Mom's heart, and I understood that she needed to talk about it. Those conversations helped me understand her deep affection for her father, a man with many flaws but a tender heart. She spoke of her daddy often in the manner of a five-year-old.

I had not anticipated what a gift those daily conversations would be. I had expected the adjustments and the sacrifices of caregiving, but the joy caught me completely off guard. I had always loved my mother, but knowing her more completely only made me love her more.

Our days were slow but pleasant. And yet, the new living arrangement represented a significant loss of freedom for me. I had always been fiercely independent and, until my sudden job loss, had milked every minute for all it was worth. Now I was operating at an octogenarian's pace. Everything took ten times longer. I remember flopping down on the sofa at noon, exhausted. It had taken all morning to get Mom fed, showered, and dressed. In many ways, I was reliving first-time motherhood with a newborn.

In hindsight, I didn't cope with those changes as well as I thought I had. I certainly didn't resent Mom for the changes because I genuinely loved caring for her and making her comfortable. But to acknowledge the simultaneous feeling of personal loss, and yes, grief, would have left me feeling guilty and selfish. So I didn't.

7
Finding Purpose

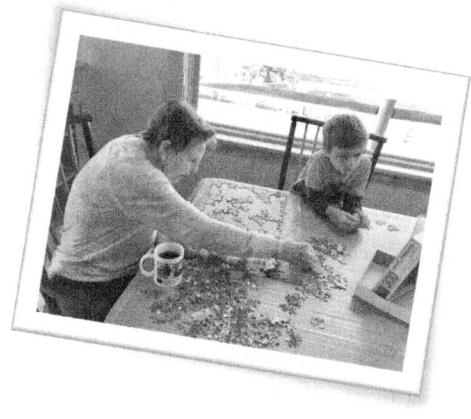

I AM MY MOTHER'S DAUGHTER. Mom was no more content being a couch potato than I was. She had taught a woman's Sunday School class for years, led countless Bible studies in her home, prepared funeral dinners, and hosted fancy tea parties with her girlfriends. The kitchen was her happy place, and she found fulfillment in serving others. Over the years, her friends had leaned on her for comfort, encouragement, prayer, and wise counsel.

During her time at College View, Mom had participated in a women's Bible study. The group graciously welcomed her continued participation even after she moved in with us. I took her every week for about a year, but it gradually became too difficult for her to follow the discussion. Thus ended her only social activity.

I could leave Mom alone for short periods of time—a hair appointment or a grocery run—but for anything longer, I needed to find someone to stay with her. Mom's long-term care policy reimbursed us for the cost of hiring respite caregivers, as long as the caregivers were not family members. I had no idea where to find the help we needed, so I tapped into my friend network and discovered that two of my friends' moms were very willing to help.

Toni and Barb, both in their seventies, became Mom's respite caregivers and dear friends. Once a week, I spent the afternoon at a coffeeshop while Toni or Barb stayed with Mom. Occasionally, Roger and I would make a trip to see our kids and grandkids, and Toni would stay several days with Mom. What a relief to know she was in good hands, and actually having a great time, in our absence!

Friendship is such a blessing, dividing our sorrows and multiplying our joys. With common cultural touch points, Mom and her caregivers talked nonstop for hours. We paid Toni and Barb well, but they grew to love Mom so much that the compensation didn't matter nearly as much as the friendship.

Jigsaw puzzles became our chief activity. Mom preferred the extra-large pieces with no more than 300 pieces. We worked at least two each week and would pass them on to the residents at College View when we were done.

There was a sweet spot with puzzles, where the challenge was difficult but attainable. For Mom, the sweet spot shifted over time. I learned that I needed to work with her closely at the start of a puzzle, helping focus her attention on the outside frame first, and then sorting the pieces by color. As the picture came into focus and fewer pieces remained, I could leave her to work on it alone.

Over time, however, puzzles became increasingly difficult for her. An activity that had once served as hours of happy entertainment eventually became a source of frustration. We had to limit the amount of time to keep it fun. She would often insist that a piece went in a place it obviously did not, and she did not appreciate our efforts to dissuade her.

Aside from puzzles, books were Mom's greatest love. With her bum hand, it was easier for her to read on a Kindle than to hold a book. That worked for a while, but technology of any kind began to overwhelm her. Eventually, we put the Kindle away and found ways to help her hold a book.

We got her a library card and checked out a new stack of books every other week. She enjoyed browsing the shelves and had strong opinions about what she did and did not want to read. Cozy mysteries were her favorite. She loved Agatha Christie, except the Hercule Poirot series, which she despised! If I held up a book whose cover suggested a sappy romance, she responded with a wrinkled nose, pursed lips, and a firm "No, thank you."

With her limited mobility and nearly useless left hand, it was difficult for Mom to help with much around the house. But oh, how she wanted to help! One day, she mentioned that my oak buffet looked terribly dry. Didn't I know that I should be treating it regularly with lemon oil? No, actually, it had never crossed my mind. But I happened to have some lemon oil (who knows why?), so I gave her a rag and turned her loose. You would think I had given her an expensive gift such was her delight. It became a standing joke. Whenever she was bored, one of us would break out the lemon oil. My furniture had never been so hydrated.

Roger was more sensitive to Mom's need to be productive than I was. For two years, he sold an elderly man's lifetime collection of license plates and miscellaneous automotive items on eBay, working on commission. With her background in antiques, Mom loved participating in this venture. Sometimes Roger would have boxes of small items, like hundreds of radiator emblems, that needed to be cleaned. He would set Mom up at the dining room table and let her clean, polish, and sort to her heart's content.

With four children, eleven grandchildren, and an ever-growing number of great-grandchildren, Mom kept Hallmark in business. She took birthday cards seriously, selecting just the right one for each adult and child.

She poured similar effort into her Christmas card list, the holidays being the only time she kept in touch with many cherished friends. I helped her write a Christmas letter and addressed the envelopes. She signed her name and wrote a personal note at the bottom of each letter. So many people she loved lived far away, and she delighted in sending and receiving cards.

Mom maintained a sunny disposition most of the time, so it surprised me one day when she looked across the living room at me and said, "I just feel so bad."

"Mom! What's wrong? What's making you feel bad?" I asked.

"I'm not doing anything to help anybody. I so want to help people, but I can't do anything. I'm just useless."

My sweet mama had lost so much, but being deprived of the ability to serve other people might have been the most painful loss of all. It cut to the core of her identity.

We put our heads together and came up with a plan. Three of my former colleagues had young children, and I was sensitive to the incessant demands on working parents.

"Mom, what if we make dinner one night each month for Rachel, Jen, and Fredrick?" I suggested. We would plan the menus together, and she could help prepare the food. I suggested that she might also like to find a scripture verse to send with the meal.

Her reaction: pure joy. She spent an entire day thumbing through her Bible and making a list of encouraging scriptures. When Jen stopped by to pick up her dinner the first time, she read the verse Mom had selected for her and tears rolled down her cheeks. What a God moment for us all. Jen told me recently that she still has that scripture verse taped to her mirror.

It took a lot of effort for me to help Mom feel productive and useful. Often, my bucket of ideas ran dry, and I grew weary of the work. But moments like the one with Jen made it all worthwhile. We are God-designed to need human connection, and what felt like busy work turned out to be my most important contribution to Mom's happiness and well-being.

While Mom had the bulk of my attention, I tried to maintain some separation, pursuing my own interests. I met friends for coffee, went to a yoga class once a week, and took Rawley for afternoon walks.

My blog was my primary outlet. Toni came to sit with Mom on Thursday afternoons while I went to a coffeeshop to write. But any serious writing requires sustained blocks of time and attention. I had neither. I dabbled, posting infrequently, always longing for something more substantive.

Roger and I went to church together and participated in a small group with church friends. Our primary social activity was a standing Friday night date, playing cards with another couple. We always met at our house, and Mama watched *Perry Mason* while we played. Not exactly living the high life, but it was something.

8
Managing Healthcare

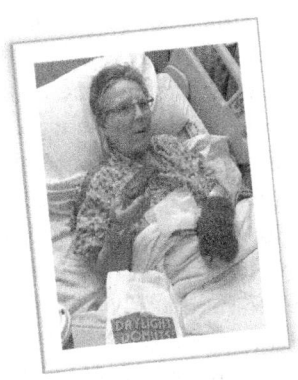

BEGINNING WITH MY FIRST DEER-in-the-headlights moment with the paramedic in Colorado, I had a lot to learn about managing Mom's healthcare. The first order of business when she moved to Missouri was finding a doctor who took her insurance. She had a Medicare Advantage plan, sometimes called a Medicare Part C plan, which meant absolutely nothing to me.

I had to quickly come up to speed on Medicare terminology. I learned that a Medicare Advantage plan is an alternative to traditional Medicare, offered by private insurers. While there are several differences, two became important to us at different times.

First, coverage is limited to a network of providers within a service area, which meant we had to pay out-of-pocket when Mom needed medical care during a trip to Wyoming. Second, it does not cover nursing home care. When she needed those services, we switched to a traditional Medicare plan, and it was no problem.

Mom's health history was complicated. In addition to her stroke, she'd had four hip surgeries, a broken ankle (repaired with steel plates), a hysterectomy, pneumonia, and a pulmonary embolism. Fortunately, she didn't have cancer or diabetes, but we checked the box for high blood pressure, high cholesterol, osteoporosis, hypothyroidism, and chronic kidney disease. Soon we could add atherosclerosis and pleural effusion.

One of the most frustrating aspects of the American healthcare system is that it operates in silos and seems to thrive on duplication of effort. Even within a network of providers who share computer systems, each provider requires a paper copy of the same information in the computer. These inefficiencies are baffling to anyone with a business background, and yet they persist.

Before long, I started taking a small three-ring binder with me to all her appointments. It contained:

- A complete medical history with dates of diagnoses and surgeries
- A current list of medications and supplements with dosages
- A list of drug allergies
- Legal documents, including an advance directive, a general power of attorney, and a healthcare power of attorney

I kept her Medicare ID, insurance card, and photo ID in her wallet, but those could just have easily been added to the notebook. Not only was the notebook handy for our routine doctor visits, but I also left it with Mom's respite caregivers in case of emergency. Eventually, I carried most of the documents digitally on my phone.

In addition to navigating the healthcare system, I had to learn how to be Mom's best advocate. Some doctors tend to be quick to order imaging tests or prescribe drugs. I asked a lot of questions, and sometimes we chose a lesser course of action.

For example, when Mom dislocated her hip again, a year after moving to Joplin, the orthopedic doctor was willing to try a surgical corrective action. But "try" was not the word I was looking for. I knew how difficult surgery would be for Mom, and we opted to continue with the brace instead. Eventually, the hip got strong enough that she no longer needed the brace. Of course, it could have gone the other way, and she might have ended up in emergency surgery again. But I had made a judgment call with the best information available. The entirety of my medical training came from Google. I second-guessed myself a lot.

Our culture leans heavily on pharmaceuticals, and at an advanced age, most people have several conditions to treat. In Mom's case, we systematically began reducing her drugs. Did she really need the osteoporosis medication? No. We stopped it. She also took a lot of vitamins and homeopathic pills, like fish oil tablets that she believed helped her brain. We gradually eliminated or reduced those.

Another decision came when Mom's dementia began to worsen rapidly. Sensing my anxiety, our family physician, Dr. Thomas, offered a new medication we could try. When I questioned the likelihood of it really alleviating Mom's symptoms, he admitted that it would not help her regain any of the lost ground. It may slow down the acceleration, he said, but he wasn't overly confident it would have even that marginal benefit. I understood that he was giving me all the possible options, and I appreciated his honest assessment of the drug's potential value for mom. He generally supported my "less is best" approach to medications, and in keeping with that philosophy, I declined to try the new drug.

Dr. Thomas and his staff interacted graciously with Mom, speaking to her directly and listening well. They gave her respect and dignity. Still, she didn't always give accurate information. As he conversed with Mom, Dr. Thomas mastered the art of the quick side glance, taking in my raised eyebrow or subtle head shake to provide additional context.

I longed to have a frank conversation with him about Mom's progressing dementia, to be able to ask my questions and get his professional opinion about what to expect next. But Mom was always present, and if I had excused her from the room for a few minutes, she would have felt I was withholding something from her. In the end, I chose to err on the side of respecting Mom's feelings. I would rely on Dr. Google for those questions.

When Mom began having some unusual symptoms that didn't point to any clear source, Dr. Thomas ordered a CT scan of her torso. The scan revealed a mass of some kind in her mid-section, but it wasn't clear exactly where it was. Maybe on the adrenal gland? The radiologist couldn't tell, but sure enough, there was something in there that shouldn't be.

Apparently, the accidental discovery of a mysterious mass is not uncommon. They even have a name for it: an *incidentaloma*. Who knew?

We decided to wait and monitor the situation. In two months, we repeated the scan and the mass had grown slightly.

At that point, we had two options: leave it alone and continue to monitor it or do a biopsy. In hindsight, we should have left it alone. After all, regardless of what a biopsy showed, we had already decided we would not do surgery. But getting an answer seemed important at the time, so we scheduled the biopsy.

The day of the procedure, they wheeled Mom down a hallway, and I waited in the waiting room. Sometime later the doctor came out and briefed me. He said that as he was getting ready to start the procedure, he had realized that there was no way to get the needle into the mass without piercing the pleural lining, the area around the lung. Anesthesia had yet to be administered, so he had talked to Mom about the risks involved and obtained her consent to continue. But he didn't talk to me! If I had been informed, we might have declined the procedure, but it was too late by the time I knew.

Legally, the doctor had every right to act on Mom's consent. As far he could tell, she was of sound mind. In the five minutes he spent with her, he didn't recognize her limited ability to process the important decision he was asking her to make. But he knew I was in the waiting room, and he could have taken a few more minutes to bring me into the conversation.

After all that, the biopsy had been unsuccessful. They had been unable to obtain a tissue sample. The doctor described the mass as "sponge-like" and mostly air. Very weird, but he felt confident it was benign.

I was tucking Mom in a few nights later when she complained of a heaviness in her chest. She had pain in her arm and said it felt like an elephant was sitting on her chest. Alarmed, I told her we needed to go to the emergency room. She emphatically disagreed.

"Mom, what you're describing sounds like a heart attack," I explained. "We really need to get it checked out right away."

"No," she said again. "I'm not going to the hospital. We are all going to bed, and we'll see how I feel in the morning."

Against my better judgment, I kissed her goodnight. It was her call, and I needed to respect it, even if I didn't agree.

The next morning, she was worse, and we immediately went to the ER. After hours of waiting and testing, we learned she had a pleural effusion. Fluid had built up around her lungs as a result of the biopsy. She was miserable.

She spent three days in the hospital, over Christmas, and Elaine came down to be with us. They drained more than a liter of fluid off her lungs, then did a chest X-ray and another CT scan. The new CT showed that the mass had dramatically increased in size.

Now the hospitalist read through the reports and, given the growth in the mass, determined that the mass almost certainly was an aggressive cancer. Even without a pathology report, he felt confident in his diagnosis, and we left the hospital with instructions to begin hospice services.

Mom was calm and pragmatic about the diagnosis, and we started thinking about how we wanted to spend her last few months of life. We got set up with hospice, and they began coming by a couple of times a week. She was not displaying any of the normal symptoms of someone with aggressive cancer, but the hospice professionals talked us through what to expect… eventually.

Those months of health crisis prompted some critical conversations. As Mom's designated power of attorney for healthcare decisions, I felt the weight of responsibility. The night she had refused to let me take her to the hospital when I thought she might have been having a heart attack left me rattled. When the crisis had subsided, I probed more deeply about her healthcare wishes.

"Mom, I'm the person who will make healthcare decisions for you if you are ever unable to make them yourself," I said. "That responsibility feels more grave after what we've just been through, and I need to make sure I understand what you want."

I reminded her of our conversation the night before she ended up in the hospital when she had described symptoms similar to a heart attack.

"Do you remember what you were thinking that night?" I asked.

"I just didn't want to go to the hospital," she said.

I probed further, asking her to imagine how the scenario might have played out if she really had been having a heart attack. She could have died right there in her bed.

"Were you telling me that you would *not* want me to intervene if you were having a heart attack, or did you just think it wasn't really that serious?" I asked.

"I guess I just thought it wasn't really that serious. I'm not sure."

That's what I had assumed, I told her, since I knew she generally favored a "wait and see" approach. But I needed to clarify her wishes to be certain I was doing what she really wanted.

I asked her to imagine the same scenario happening again. She feels terrible and it could be a heart attack, but she tells me she wants to wait until morning.

"Now that I know you really don't want me to let you die in your bed, I might very well override your protestations and insist we go to the hospital. And you'd be okay with that, right?" I asked.

"Yes, I would want you to use your judgment if you think it's that serious," she replied.

We talked about other scenarios that may arise and went through the details of the healthcare directive. I knew Mom's ability to process such weighty decisions was declining rapidly, and I was relieved to have a frank conversation while she was still in full possession of her mental faculties.

In April, we repeated the CT scan to discover the mass was dramatically smaller! Dr. Thomas concluded that she didn't have cancer after all. Whatever the mass was, it had reacted to the biopsy by swelling. That was all. It had just been one of those weird things that doctors can't explain.

Relieved, we took a deep breath and reoriented our minds to a longer period of time with Mom. How long? Of course, no one ever knows the number of their days, but it now looked very likely that 2017 would *not* be the last year of her life. Mom's health had been tenuous for years. We would take whatever time we could get.

9
Terminal Living

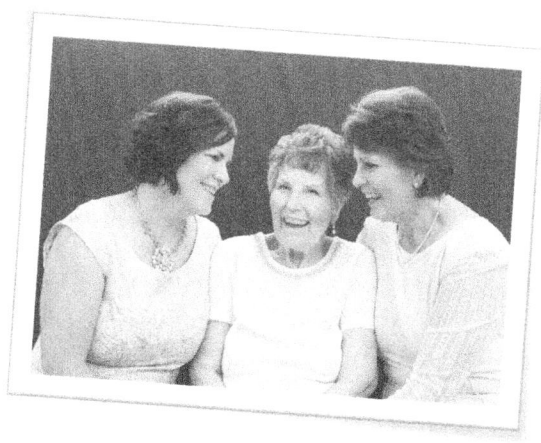

DURING THE TIME WE BELIEVED Mom's life might be measured in months instead of years, I felt a renewed sense of urgency. That feeling persisted even after we learned the diagnosis was a mistake. More than just making plans for things we wanted to do, I saw each day as a gift.

Before we got the news of the misdiagnosis, I was scrolling through Facebook one day and stopped at some stunning photos of one of my friends. Mitzi Starkweather, a local photographer, had posted the photos to advertise her portrait business.

I'm one of the least likely people to seek out professional photos, but I started thinking about what a fun experience that might be for Mom. I called Elaine and floated the idea of mother-daughter photos. We talked through the issues—the cost, Mom's physical limitations, potential scheduling challenges, the travel for Elaine. Could we pull it off? The thought of having a beautiful portrait of our mama provided powerful incentive.

I called Mitzi to get the details and told her our reason for getting the photos and our concerns about Mom's limited mobility. Mitzi reassured me we could take as much time as we needed. We booked a date in February, and Elaine made plans to come down that weekend.

For the Luxe photo experience, we would need several outfits each, including something fancy in white and in black. We didn't own anything fancy, but I made a trip to Dillard's and came home with some possibilities. The black dress I chose for Mom was a tea-length sheath with a lace overlay bodice that boasted three tiers of flapper fringe. Mom lit up when she saw it and giggled like a schoolgirl.

Mitzi operated her fledgling business out of her home. When we arrived for our photo shoot, I nearly panicked when I saw the steps we would have to navigate to get to the front door. Oof. Somehow, eventually, we got Mom into the house. We were anxious anyway, and starting the day with that challenge put us all a little on edge. But Mitzi made us feel comfortable, and one by one, we took turns having our hair and make-up done by her stylist.

As Mitzi took both individual and group photos, I couldn't stop staring at Mom. She was so beautiful! The stylist who did her hair and makeup had known just how to make her natural beauty shine. It felt like we were having our own dress-up party, like little girls playing in their mother's closet. Truly a magical day.

Two weeks later, the photos were ready and we stared in disbelief. Mitzi had made us look like movie stars. We laughingly called them our "glamour shots."

There were so many stunning photos of Mom that we had a hard time choosing only a few. The ones with the flapper dress were favorites, of course, but another of her wearing a lavender jacket and black lace top was my favorite. She was looking into the camera with a tender, soft expression, and her eyes just shone. I knew this would be the photo we'd someday use for her funeral.

Our Luxe photo shoot with Mitzi was impractical on so many levels. Difficult. Extravagant. We could have found any number of reasons to talk ourselves out of it, but I'm so glad we didn't. Sometimes it's the right call to indulge in a whim and make a little magic.

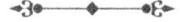

From the beginning, I was determined that Mom was going to live life to the fullest. Each day we faced the reality that someday she would be confined to her bed or her chair, but that day was not today. No, as long as it was physically possible for her to move, we were going to move.

One of the first things we did after she got settled in Joplin was trade her car for a newer model. Car shopping with Mom proved challenging, but we quickly identified the Ford Edge as the model we wanted. It was just the right height to enable her to sit and swing her legs in. The seats were comfortable—and heated!—and it had easy-access cargo space for her walker and wheelchair.

Once we settled on the model, it was just a matter of finding the right one. Call it good fortune or a divine blessing, we found exactly what we wanted at a fair price within a few days. From the day I drove it home until her last ride in it, she never failed to exclaim how much she loved her car. Good thing, because we put some miles on it.

We made several long road trips but also found many adventures within a two-hour driving radius. In the spring, we celebrated nature's beauty with a trip to Dogwood Canyon in Branson at the height of dogwood season. Or we perused crafts and ate funnel cakes at the Dogwood Festival in Siloam Springs, Arkansas. In summer, I took her to a local blueberry patch, set her bucket on her walker, and let her pick. One day, we packed two wiggly grandsons and a picnic and headed to Springfield to visit the Wonders of Wildlife aquarium.

Autumn in the Ozarks meant trips to the local pumpkin patch to fill the car with mums, pumpkins, and gourds. It was also the prime season for community celebrations, and Mama loved a good bluegrass festival. We wrung delight from every stage of these little trips—the anticipation, the fun at the moment, and the memories afterward.

We loved adding Mom to our family traditions. One of our favorites was "Camp Joplin," a week each summer when our grandchildren came to visit, without their parents. We packed the week with fun activities—trips to the creek to catch minnows, making tie-dye T-shirts, hiking and birdwatching, art projects, backyard water gun wars, and trips to amusement parks.

To incorporate Mom into Camp Joplin, we tapped into one of her superpowers—making dill pickles. At ages eight, six, and five, the kids were all in on this project. Following a quick trip to the farmer's market to secure the necessary cucumbers, dill, and garlic, they donned aprons and assumed their stations.

The youngest took charge of the wash station. Standing on a chair at the kitchen sink, she scrubbed every cucumber until it met Mom's standard. The other two peeled garlic cloves and snipped dill blooms, then carefully placed them in the bottom of sterilized jars. The oldest measured the salt and vinegar into a pot, then stirred it on the stove until it came to a boil under Mom's watchful eye. Packing the cucumbers into the jars turned into a contest, but the youngest had the clear advantage with her little hands and fierce determination.

By the time we lifted the finished quarts out of the canning kettle, Mom was ready for her recliner and the kids were elated by their accomplishment. It will forever be one of the kids' favorite Camp Joplin memories, documented, of course, in photo books.

Every summer, we made at least one big trip, usually to Wyoming to see my brothers and their families. On the way, we stopped in Colorado to visit Mom's dear friends.

One year, we rented a gorgeous cabin in Cody, Wyoming, for a family reunion. Located on the south fork of the Shoshone River, the cabin had its own private trout pond where the little kids spent many happy hours.

After leaving Cody, we drove through Yellowstone and spent the night in Grand Teton National Park. Our cabin at Colter Bay proved a logistical challenge for Mom's wheelchair but nothing two strong men couldn't manage. We stopped for numerous photo ops in front of the majestic Tetons, then continued our trip south, stopping in Pinedale, Wyoming, where my grandmother was born. Mom still had cousins there, and we spent a day catching up with them before starting the long trip back to Missouri.

It would be hard to overstate Mom's joy at being back in her beloved Rocky Mountains. Each place along our route that summer held special memories for her, and she relished the chance to step back in time. The trip was arduous for all of us, but her enraptured smiles in every photo made it worthwhile.

The next summer, we rented a house in Dubois, Wyoming. Instead of us making the rounds to see everyone in Casper, we let the family come to us. Over a three-week period, we entertained a steady stream of family, including our Texas clan. Once again, we celebrated July Fourth in small-town Western style with a patriotic parade, a rodeo, and fireworks. Dubois was only an hour from Grand Teton National Park, so we happily returned to the Tetons.

Hauling Mom all over God's creation this way was difficult and exhausting, but for the first several years, the benefits outweighed the costs. Mom lived for those times.

But by our last trip to Dubois, the scales had tipped. Mom was mostly miserable for those three weeks, and even time with her family could not ease her misery. She fought a urinary tract infection the whole time and found her bed impossibly uncomfortable. She did her best to power through, but she simply didn't have the physical and emotional bandwidth to handle it with her usual good grace.

I knew that, when the memory of her misery had faded in a few months, she'd start talking about the next trip to Wyoming. I drew a line in the sand on our way home and told her this was her last trip to Wyoming. I don't think she believed me at first, and sure enough, she was soon pining to go back. But I was done.

Fortunately, we had made photo books after most of those trips. When her traveling days ended, the photo books enabled her to relive each trip from her recliner. Nothing in the world mattered more to her than being with her people. She never tired of reliving those special times.

Mom went to stay with Elaine in Indiana several times, sometimes for a few weeks in the summer, and sometimes over the Thanksgiving and Christmas holidays. This allowed Roger and me a chance to go see our kids and grandkids, and it gave Mom time with Elaine's family. It was a nine-hour drive to Elaine's house, and those trips, too, became harder for all of us.

Elaine made great efforts to ensure Mom felt comfortable and welcome in her home. She bought a recliner for her and installed a handrail on her front porch to help her navigate the two steps to the front door. She converted her formal living room into Mom's bedroom, decorating it with furniture and decor from Mom's home in Colorado. Elaine paid attention to all the little details that made her feel loved, but Mom's ability to adapt to change diminished as her dementia deepened.

Fortunately, the family often came to Mom, so she could enjoy time with them from the comforts of her own home. We all had the same desire—spend as much time with Mom as possible—and everyone made sacrifices to make that happen.

And then in 2020, the COVID pandemic upended the world. In our home, dementia picked up steam at exactly the same time.

10
Walking in the Dark

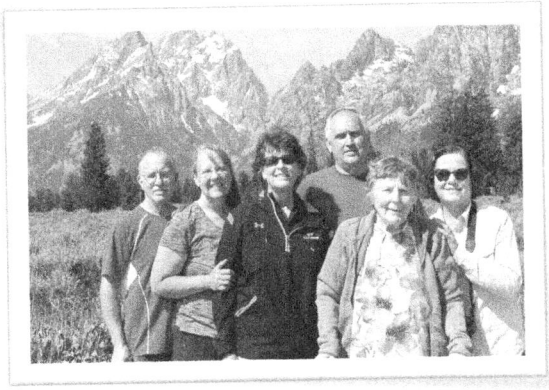

IT WOULD BE IMPOSSIBLE TO untangle the strands of Mom's worsening dementia and the consequences of isolation caused by the pandemic. Did the pandemic accelerate her symptoms? Likely not. Rather, her deepening dementia created something of a bubble, insulating her from the mental anguish the rest of the world experienced. For Roger and me, however, Mom's worsening dementia amplified the pandemic angst in our home.

Dealing with Mom's dementia was the hardest part of our caregiving journey. I kept trying to make sense of odd behaviors, kept trying to anticipate what might come next. But with its many forms and non-linear progression, dementia often defies prediction.

Mom had enjoyed a relatively stable four years in our home. We had seen early signs of dementia throughout that time—searching for words, repeating herself—but these were minor and episodic with no significant impact on our daily routine. That changed in 2020.

For those walking alongside a loved one with dementia, it can feel like traversing an unfamiliar room in the dark. Maybe our experience can serve as a flashlight. Although not a straight-line progression, here's how Mom's dementia advanced.

Cognitive Impairment

Mom spent the bulk of her days working jigsaw puzzles and reading. I would help her get started on a new puzzle, and once the frame was complete, I could leave her to work on it while I did other things. I would stop by periodically and help her with a section, but she preferred to work independently on it.

I started noticing that she would frequently try to force puzzle pieces into places they obviously did not belong. She could no longer distinguish, for example, that a piece with a horse's legs could only go one direction, with the legs pointed down. Or that a piece with a pink flower didn't go in the blue sky.

I tried to help her reason through why a piece didn't go in a certain place. I wondered if it could be her vision.

"Mom, let's look at this piece. What is it?"

"I don't know."

"Well, to me it looks like the horse's legs," I said, pointing to the picture on the box. "If that's what it is, where do you think it might go?"

She might find the general area of the puzzle, but she couldn't process that the legs needed to be pointed downward. Her vision may have been part of the problem, but it became evident that the bigger issue was cognitive.

If I left her to work on a puzzle independently, she quickly became frustrated. Instead, I worked with her and set time limits to minimize her distress. Roger brought some levity to the situation when he suggested he was going to get her a "puzzle hammer" for Christmas, so she could pound those pieces into submission!

Once when Mom was visiting Elaine, the two of them had just started taking a puzzle out of the box when Elaine got a phone call. She left the room to take the call and when she returned, Mom had carefully arranged all the puzzle pieces on the table—upside down. She was unable to distinguish the design side from the cardboard underside. It was a sad day.

We also learned that puzzles were not an activity she could enjoy with her great-grandchildren. When six-year-old Miles insisted, "Nana, that piece doesn't go there," Mom became exasperated. Time for a new activity.

The same thing happened with books. We went to the library every week, and she checked out three or four titles, usually cozy mysteries. I began to notice the erratic placement of her bookmark. Suddenly she was on chapter two of a book that I thought she had almost finished. It became apparent that she had no idea what she was reading and could not follow the storyline at all. She continued to "read," out of habit or denial, long past her ability to comprehend. Eventually, she gave up reading altogether.

Technology was the worst. Her Kindle, iPhone, iPad—one-by-one the frustration became unbearable for all of us. She simply could not master a simple sequence of steps no matter how many times we practiced it. She took this loss harder than the others and probably felt that I was being mean to remove them. I struggled with the decision, knowing she wouldn't understand, but I had reached my limit.

Mental Anguish

I grew up in non-liturgical faith traditions, so I've only recently discovered Compline, the night prayer from the Anglican *Book of Common Prayer*. It begins this way:

> *Keep watch, dear Lord, with those who work, or watch, or weep this night, and give your Angels charge over those who sleep.*

At first blush, it seems that sleep should be a period of peace and safety. Why do we need angelic protection, especially at night? Because at night, problems loom larger. The subconscious mind trots out fears and mistakes and old wounds. Our minds are particularly vulnerable at night. When the world is quiet, we are alone and our brains are unfettered from conscious thought. I've experienced it myself, and Mom experienced it more often with the progression of dementia.

In the early years of her time with us, I'd watch her wake up after a difficult night and see her walk herself through negative feelings to reach emotional equanimity. A woman of steadfast faith, she drew from a deep well of memorized scripture and approached the throne of grace with confidence. In recent years, however, sometimes the remnants of a difficult night lingered past noon. She needed to talk it out.

The source of her mental distress was predictable: childhood hurts in her relationship with her mother and difficult seasons in her marriage to my father. She also suffered parenting guilt, especially regarding one child. While the source of her mental pain had some basis in reality, it was overblown and lacked perspective. Her mother and husband were both dead, so she had no opportunity to resolve the issues that robbed her of sleep. We would talk through them, pray through them, and put them into a larger, more grace-filled perspective. With regard to her parenting guilt, she could address those issues directly, and she did.

Hallucinations

Years earlier, when Mom was recovering from her stroke, she had experienced hallucinations. On one occasion, she had seen a baby in the middle of the living room floor. On another, she had witnessed vicious, snarling dogs. At the time, her doctor had put her on a seizure medication, but Mom hated the side effects and eventually stopped taking it. She had experienced no more hallucinations after that brief season.

They returned with her dementia. Sometimes they occurred in the middle of the day, but more often at night, and they involved her senses of smell and sound, not just sight.

On one occasion, when she was at Elaine's house, Mom called out to Elaine in the middle of the night. Elaine flew down the stairs, thinking maybe she had fallen out of bed. Instead, she was safely ensconced in her quilts, but she asked Elaine if she would please get all those birds off the ceiling. Even with the lights on, Elaine confessed she couldn't see the birds, so she asked Mom to show her where they were. Mom pointed to the corner. Elaine got a folding chair and a broom, carefully sweeping that corner until Mom said they were all gone.

Because her hallucinations frequently happened at night, it was easiest to label them as vivid dreams, even though she insisted she was awake. I greeted her one morning and found her in a panic because she smelled gas. Another time she heard a group of men talking in the yard outside her window, and she thought they were Roger's friends who had come to pick him up for some activity. Only it was 4:00 a.m., and there were no men and no activity. One morning she reported that our grandsons had been playing noisily in the living room and wondered why they were being loud so early in the morning.

The way we handled these episodes of alternate reality depended on how she felt about what she thought she had seen or heard or smelled. When she woke up worried because she smelled gas, I walked with her through the house to see if she was still smelling it. Eventually, she acknowledged that whatever she had smelled was gone and we were safe.

If the episode was more benign—curiosity aroused by the men in the yard at 4:00 a.m. or exasperation at the noisy little boys in the living room—we explained the episode as a dream. I wanted to acknowledge the realness of what she had experienced but also gently bring her back into reality. Those noisy little boys in the living room? We laughed that Miles and Graham had been so rowdy the last time they were here, she was still dreaming about their rambunctiousness!

She accepted these explanations with skepticism. The morning she heard the men in the yard, she had reluctantly agreed it must have been a dream, but we had to process it all over again after lunch. The event was so real in her mind that she could not reconcile it with the reality we presented her. It troubled her. We sought to reassure her and divert her attention to something more pleasant.

Disorientation

We first started noticing Mom's disorientation when she was away from home. Even if it was a familiar place, like Elaine's house, she would get confused navigating from one room to the next. It was understandable in places we visited for our summer trips, like the cabins in Cody and Dubois. But then it started happening at home.

Mom's bedroom was just off the living room, and her recliner was a few steps from her bedroom door. When she wanted to go to her bedroom, she would often stand in front of her recliner, clutching her walker, unsure of which direction to turn. Her bedroom door was a mere three feet to her right, the same path she had navigated for five years, but she could no longer remember.

Loss of Mobility

Since her stroke years before, Mom had struggled with balance and mobility. Thanks to excellent therapists and her own determination, she had regained most of the left-side deficit caused by her stroke, but when she was fatigued, the left leg didn't always cooperate.

As her dementia worsened, that leg sometimes stopped listening to her brain. She would try to lift her foot, to no avail.

Once at Elaine's house, they were trying to get her through the front door, which required her to lift her foot a couple of inches to clear the threshold. She could not do it. The more she tried, the more frustrated she became. And then my brother-in-law, Dan, hit upon a brilliant idea.

"Norma, I know how to get that leg to move," he declared. He pulled out his phone, did a quick Internet search, and then proceeded to play the "Beer Barrel Polka." Sure enough, that favorite song from her dancing days rewired the circuit between brain and leg, and she lifted her foot over the threshold with ease!

We deployed the "Beer Barrel Polka" technique many times after that. Sometimes it worked, sometimes it didn't. We could usually avoid the issue by using the wheelchair instead of the walker, but sometimes, like stepping into the shower, getting the leg to cooperate was our only option.

Even when the leg was working, she started to lose her balance more. On two occasions, she managed to topple over with her walker, scaring us silly. We lived in fear of a broken hip.

Rising Anxiety

As her dementia worsened, Mom became anxious if I was out of her sight. The days were gone when I could make a quick trip to the grocery store or yoga class.

I have a small office area on our upstairs landing, and one day I spent a couple of hours at my desk working on taxes. I told her I was going upstairs for a bit. Our house was so small, I was literally only a few feet away. But she couldn't see me and she immediately forgot what I had told her. When I came downstairs two hours later, she was sitting in her recliner, crying.

"Oh, there you are!" she exclaimed. "I've been so worried something happened to you, and I didn't know who was going to take care of me!"

It broke my heart to see her so upset, and it was undeniable proof that we had entered a new chapter. From that point forward, Roger and I couldn't both be gone for any length of time. Fortunately, the pandemic had postponed our church and small group meetings, and we could easily work around the necessary errands. But even when I was home, I couldn't be out of her sight for more than a few minutes or she became very anxious.

Loss of Appetite

In early 2021, I noticed Mom was barely touching her food. Previously, she had kept a healthy appetite and relished three meals a day. Now I found her sneaking her oatmeal to the dog. Sometimes, she only nibbled at dinner, even when it was one of her favorite foods. When I asked her about it, she replied with a shrug, "I'm just not hungry." What started as an occasional disinterest in food progressed rapidly until she was hardly eating at all. Once again, we were entering new territory.

Dr. Thomas recommended a cognitive assessment for Mom. By that time, I didn't need an assessment to tell me what I was seeing, but I knew it might be an important piece of data for the future. I sat beside Mom while a kind nurse walked through a series of basic questions.

What year is it?

What season is it?
Where do you live?
How many children do you have?
What are your children's names?
Who is the President?

About twenty-five questions total, and she didn't get any of them right, including my name. Sometimes she answered with great confidence, like when she declared she lived in Cincinnati. No. She lived in Joplin, Missouri.

At the end of the exam, she looked expectantly at the nurse and said, "Well, how'd I do?"

"Not very well," the nurse replied with a sympathetic smile. "It seems you are not remembering well. Does it bother you that you can't remember things?"

Mom thought for a minute and then answered, "No, not really."

I had to smile. That's the thing about dementia. Those who have it are not the ones who suffer most; it's the people who love them.

Some patients experience dramatic personality changes with dementia. Fortunately, Mom never got cranky or irritable. In fact, she got sweeter.

Eventually, we noticed a certain absence in her demeanor, a lack of spark. She felt distant. I could tell how hard she was working to understand me when I was talking to her, and often the shadow of a question mark lingered on her face, even as she nodded her head to indicate she understood. Daily life, as quiet as it was, took so much effort. She seemed worn out most of the time.

Yet every single day, she told me how much she appreciated us and how happy and safe she felt in our home. She acknowledged the sacrifices we made for her, and she was deeply grateful. We, too, were grateful. And worn out.

I had no crystal ball, but I knew we were on the brink of a change. From time to time, I had talked with Mom about various scenarios when her health declined. I knew she wanted to live with us until she died, but I also knew that might become impossible. So we talked openly about what scenario might make it impossible for us to continue to care for her.

"Mom, you know I have a bad back, and if it ever gets to the point where you can't walk, I won't be able to lift you," I said.

She nodded. "I know. I wouldn't want you to hurt yourself."

"But I promise we will always take care of you, even if we eventually need the help of trained professionals. You know that, right?"

"Yes, I know."

What I didn't mention, what kept me awake at night, was knowing the nursing homes were closed to family members in response to COVID. The prospect of her being under someone else's care and me being unable to see her was a future too terrible to ponder.

I did a lot of praying and encouraged her to walk laps around the kitchen island several times a day to keep her legs strong. It began to look like a toss-up who would buckle first, her or me.

11
Caregiver in Crisis

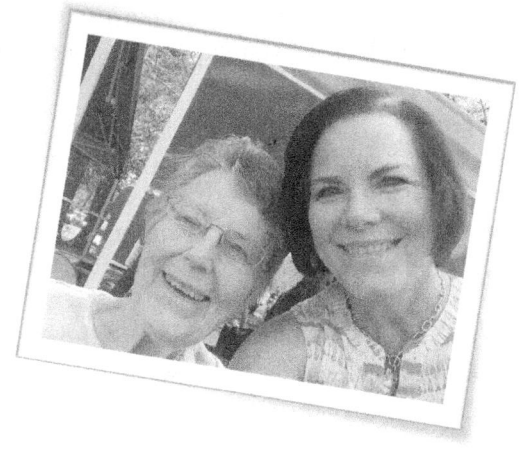

DURING THE FIRST YEAR OF the pandemic as Mom's decline accelerated, I began to struggle as well. Only I couldn't see it. We spiraled downward in tandem, too fixated on day-to-day survival to see the trend.

The innocent optimism of the 2020 new year hadn't even lasted until the first daffodil bloom. By March 2020, COVID-19 held the entire world in apocalyptic terror. While our financial portfolios tanked, we donned face masks, dodged strangers, and wiped our groceries with Clorox wipes.

In the early months of the pandemic, home felt like a cozy refuge. Apparently, the whole country simultaneously felt the urge to bake bread, making yeast impossible to find on grocery store shelves. We hunkered down, watched old movies, and told ourselves it would all be over in a few months.

For the rest of the year, we watched news reports of crying nurses, families holding up signs at nursing home windows, and mobile morgues being set up in hospital parking lots. We canceled trips and holiday celebrations, attended church in our pajamas from the living room, and maintained six feet of social distance from anyone other than family. We lived in a perpetual crouch.

At the same time, America faced a political firestorm fueled by falsehoods, corruption, and bare-knuckled vitriol that divided friends and families into warring tribes. Any hope for relief after the November election quickly evaporated as the rhetoric and lies ratcheted to dangerous levels. The phrase "Constitutional crisis" wore out from overuse.

During this global and national hurricane of misery, we dealt with personal misery inside our own four walls. As Mom's dementia progressed, she needed more and more care and could no longer entertain herself with any activity. I sat with her for a good portion of every day, and we watched excessive amounts of news. Roger and I became distant, our relationship strained by the long drain on our resources, political differences, and a lack of time together.

I found myself taking at least two naps a day. Thanks to yoga pants, I could largely ignore the extra pounds I had gradually gained. I couldn't muster enthusiasm for writing, so my blog languished.

By late 2020, I knew I was in trouble. Roger had known it many months earlier. My heart was in turmoil. My body was tired. My mind wrestled with fear. And I felt very alone.

I sorted through the wreckage in the only way I knew, by writing the chaos into some sort of order. My journal entries paint a clear picture of the sources of my angst.

The Long Goodbye

I had lost my dad suddenly, with no warning and no opportunity to say goodbye. Now I was losing my mother piece by piece, over slow years, as that demon dementia quietly erased her in front of my very eyes.

When I looked back at selfies I had taken with Mom in the early years of her living with us, I was shocked by the contrast. Her bright eyes and easy smile exuded a child-like joy and spirit of adventure. In spite of the challenge of her limited mobility, we had made numerous day trips to nature centers, craft fairs, and music events. She had never turned down a shopping trip to Hobby Lobby or an invitation to wander the aisles of an antiques mall. Now those activities held no interest for her.

One by one, she had lost most every delight. The jigsaw puzzles that had once happily occupied hours of her day now threw her into anxious confusion. It was the same for books. She had given up even the pretense of reading, as words on a page made no sense. Only music still brought her joy. With her favorite Daniel O'Donnell CD playing, she would attempt to color in her coloring book. But what color should she use for the flower, she would ask. And what about the tree? It was all so confusing. Too many choices. Finally, she would put the pencils down and just listen to the music.

We used to chat like girlfriends. I could tell her my struggles or discuss a book I found inspiring. She would often reflect on difficult periods of her life and talk about how God had grown her faith during those struggles. Conversation was difficult now. Whereas she had first struggled to find the right word, now she often struggled to process the thought behind the word.

I missed my mom. She was right there in her recliner, and yet she wasn't. I found myself taking mental Polaroids, documenting small joys I knew would soon be gone.

Her sweet smile when I tucked her in at night.

The way her face lit up when I opened her bedroom door in the morning and she would say, "Oh, I'm so happy to see you."

The way she discovered her rooster cup collection on the kitchen windowsill every morning, as if for the first time.

Her gasps of delight upon spotting a cardinal or blue jay on the bird feeder.

Her insistence that she had never seen a sky so blue as today, a sky that could only be described as "Wyoming blue."

I struggled to hold both grief and joy, both hands open.

The Valley of the Shadow

As hard as today may be, I lived with the ever-present reality that tomorrow would be harder yet. When the Psalmist speaks of the "valley of the shadow of death," it isn't death itself that weighs on his mind. It's the looming *shadow* of death, that intangible and unassailable foe, that dogs his every step. It was coming, but not yet. Maybe today. Maybe two years from now.

The shadow of death filled me with dread, bordering on anxiety.

All signs indicated Mom's body would outlast her mind. What would that look like? I didn't know. When the light in her eyes had faded to dark, would her lungs still accept air, her throat still open for sustenance, her heart still beat out of habit? A deep anguish rose in me.

The Basin and Towel

Mom and I had traded places. She had once changed my diapers, fed me, bathed me, dressed me, tucked me in, and kept me safe. Now I did those things for her. My mothering skills were thirty-five years rusty, but I was learning again how to sleep in light-snooze mode.

In one sense, the physical care of an adult is not that different from the care of an infant or toddler. With babies, however, every day marks progress toward independence. You wipe dirty bottoms with patient resolve because potty training starts soon. Day by day, the child gains mastery—drinking from a cup, walking, feeding herself, dressing herself, and on it goes. We proudly chart every milestone in a baby book, each success a validation of our parenting.

As the "parent" of my parent, however, every day moved us one step closer to full dependence. Mom lost ground every year, every month, every week. As the physical care requirements increased, I confess to having what I called "low patience" days. My days were galaxies away from the corporate life I had once known. I was charting bowel movements instead of strategy spreadsheets. I was disinfecting the third mess of the day instead of conducting performance reviews. I was slipping out to the back porch for five minutes of fresh air instead of jetting off to China. I didn't always like the trade.

And yet, wasn't this the very essence of love? To care for someone else above yourself? Yes. Yes, of course. And my low patience days might better be described as "low Spirit" days. Days when I was living in my flesh, selfishly, rather than in the power of the Holy Spirit.

Jesus knew the insidious selfishness that lies deep in the human heart, so he gave us an object lesson we could not ignore. The One who spoke the world into existence put on a human body. Then he wrapped a towel around his waist, poured a basin of water, and kneeled to wash the dusty, grimy feet of his friends. He even washed the feet of Judas, who would soon betray him.

If I wanted to be like Jesus—and oh, how I did—the path led through a lot of unpleasant messes. I wanted desperately to be a better person than I was.

The Dream Deferred

As months stretched into years, I felt my life leaking into the beach of time. I had plans and dreams for my retirement. Writing. Traveling. Being involved with my grandchildren. Most of those dreams had been deferred until... when? I was a planner, a doer. I kept a daily planner out of habit, but the weeks held mostly blank spaces. My life looked a lot like quarantine before the pandemic, and I had only barely survived the interminable months of increased isolation.

In my raw moments with God, I found myself saying, "So... this is it then? I'm done? If so, Lord, why do I still have this burning in my bones, this bucket list of desire? And what do you want me to do with it?" The poet Langston Hughes channeled my heart in his poem "Harlem."

> *What happens to a dream deferred?*
> *Does it dry up*
> *Like a raisin in the sun?*
> *Or fester like a sore—*
> *And then run?*
> *Does it stink like rotten meat? Or crust and sugar over—*
> *Like a syrupy sweet?*
> *Maybe it just sags like a heavy load.*
> *Or does it explode?*

I knew the answer: all of the above. In an act of spiritual discipline, I was laying my dried-up dreams at His feet. They were

His to do with as He wanted. I reminded myself that He is a good, good Father, and it delights Him to give good gifts to his children.

I remembered other seasons of waiting, other dry and barren seasons, that eventually gave way to lush green pastures. I remembered how He had fed manna to the children of Israel in the desert, providing just enough sustenance for the day. Maybe they, too, had kept a planning habit He needed to break. I was tempted to fill every empty square in my planner with "manna."

One day at a time, I needed to trust Him.

The Balancing Act

I was committed to walking Mama home, making sure she would not be alone in this final valley. But I was not just a daughter. I was also a wife, a mother, a grandmother, and a friend. And I was a flesh-and-blood human who required care and maintenance. It felt like an impossible balancing act.

Our adult children were facing their own life challenges to which I could only offer moral support by phone. I desperately wanted to be more present with them. Our grandchildren were growing up, and FaceTime was a poor substitute for bear hugs and belly laughs.

And yet, even on the hardest days, I was also overwhelmed with gratitude. Thankful for the opportunity to minister to my mom. Thankful for my husband who had sacrificed without complaint. Thankful to my siblings, who provided physical and moral support. I was a mess of contradictions.

Days passed marked by reruns of *Perry Mason* and *The Lawrence Welk Show*. The house remained a balmy eighty-two degrees, but Mama would still be cold. And I was trying—really trying—to lift my hands, palms open, to receive both grief and joy.

For all my efforts to keep a positive mindset, however, I sank farther each day. I finally had to say to my husband and my siblings, "I'm not okay."

With skilled nursing facilities still on lockdown and my siblings occupied with full-time jobs, I felt stuck. I didn't want to completely pass the baton, but neither did I just need a temporary break. Roger and I discussed the possibility of a six-month rotation with Elaine.

We knew it would mean a major reordering of her life, but Roger insisted it was time.

I broached the possibility with her in a phone call and waited several days for her to think about it and call me back. When she didn't, I called her again. We talked through the difficulties and various scenarios, none of which would be simple. It seemed that every time I offered a solution, she pushed back with a reason it couldn't work. We were both frustrated, and the call ended with me hanging up on her.

Rehashing the conversation with Roger later, I was still fuming. I went full martyr mode and decided if Elaine wouldn't help, fine. I'd power through. Roger countered that Elaine was not refusing to help, that she was just having a hard time seeing a way forward. He suggested he might call her, and I made him promise he would not get in the middle of it.

But he did. Knowing how tenuous my mental health was at that time, he staged an intervention and started having conversations with my siblings, letting them know that something had to change. We could not continue our caregiving role indefinitely.

At one point, he gently said to me, "Aileen, your mom is going to die, and that relationship will end. But you may have another thirty years with your sister. Be careful."

At first, I resented his intervention. I still felt very protective of Mom, and I didn't want her to feel abandoned. It would be so hard to let go of her day-to-day care, but even I knew it needed to happen.

By early 2021, we had a plan in place. Beginning in June, Elaine and I would start taking six-month shifts as Mom's caregivers. The school where Elaine taught agreed to reduce her class load so she could be finished by 1:00 each day, and she found someone to stay with Mom in the mornings. It would not be easy, but it was the best alternative.

We planned the hand-off for the third week of June, and Roger and I started making travel plans for our six months of freedom. How we longed to see our grandchildren! The anticipation gave me mental relief, even if it was still months away.

Months earlier, I had asked my siblings to research skilled nursing facilities in their areas, in case we reached that point. The pandemic continued to rage, but we clung to hope that it would abate before we might need skilled nursing care. For all of life's uncertainty, I felt better just having a plan.

12
Passing the Baton

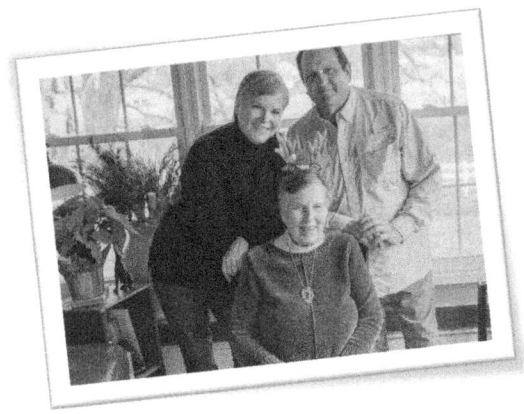

FROM MY BEDROOM UPSTAIRS, I heard her hit the floor. I ran flying down the stairs yelling, "Mama, Mama, Mama." She was crumpled next to the foot of her bed, one hand still clutching the handle of her walker. Dazed and confused, she nonetheless tried to assure me that she was not hurt. Roger helped me get her up and into her recliner, which was no small feat. We had just purchased a gait belt, one of those essential caregiver tools I had never heard of until then.

We all took a deep breath, got a cup of coffee, and settled. I continued to examine her, not convinced she was uninjured. She told me she had gotten out of bed and taken a few steps before her legs had buckled. I took her blood pressure: 87/56. Her skin was sallow and she looked absolutely wrung out.

Although convinced she had no serious injuries, the low blood pressure freaked me out. I left a message with Dr. Thomas, whose office was not yet open. As I expected, he called back and advised that we take her to the emergency room for a thorough check.

We took our time getting ready and finally checked into the packed ER just before noon. COVID cases were still rampant, and the ER staff looked worn to the nub.

For the next nine long hours, we had nothing to do but watch a parade of human misery. The security officer physically removed one irate person, whose patience had been stretched past its breaking point by an eight-hour wait. I felt his pain and appreciated the lesson in what not to do with my own frustration.

Next to the front desk, a person sat slumped in a wheelchair with a blanket over his head. The blanket covered him completely, with only his shoes visible. For hours, he did not move. Not even a twitch. *Is he dead*, I wondered in horror. I tried not to stare, but he was in my direct line of sight, and there was nothing else to distract my attention. Finally, after four hours, the blanket-covered figure shifted ever so slightly in the wheelchair, breaking the macabre spell.

At 9:30 p.m., it was finally our turn. They settled Mom onto a gurney, then wrapped her weary bones in a heated blanket.

Thank you, Jesus, for small comforts.

For the next six hours, we met a series of techs and doctors between long waits. Vital signs looked normal, blood work checked out, and x-rays showed bones still intact. At 3:30 a.m., we got the all-clear to go home.

I have no idea how I managed to get her both in and out of the car and into the house. We were both beyond exhausted when we finally collapsed into bed at 4:00 a.m. As I tucked her in, I said, "When you wake up, Mama, just wait for me to come help you, okay? We don't want to do this all over again."

"Right," she mumbled, and she was out.

I lay in bed, replaying the anxiety of the day and wondering what to do next. Elaine was due to arrive tomorrow, June 18, a few days in advance of our six-month hand-off, when Mom would go home with her. Roger and I planned to hit the road on June 24, traveling to a Dubois reunion with Roger's siblings and our kids and grandkids. My brain could no longer absorb the implications and what-ifs, and I finally fell into a deep sleep.

Like Groundhog Day, I awoke the next morning to the thud of Mom hitting the floor. Once again, I flew down the stairs, yelling "Mama, Mama, Mama!" This time she hadn't even made it two steps before collapsing. Her face a sickly yellow color, she grimaced in pain even as she assured me she was all right.

We repeated the drill with one major change. This time we called an ambulance. "Not my first rodeo," I muttered through clenched teeth as I dialed 9-1-1. Ambulance patients automatically go to the front of the line, so no matter what horrors awaited us on Day Two in the ER, it would be an improvement over Day One.

The ER staff repeated all the same tests that had been done only twelve hours before and expressed doubt that they could admit her. Her color remained that ghastly yellow, and she was sick to her stomach. Clearly, we could not take her home. At 10:00 that night, they finally admitted her to a room.

Elaine had arrived that day, but she couldn't join us in the ER due to COVID protocols. Once Mom was settled into her room, we both remained by her side. She had been administered fluids, which had eased her nausea, and some color had returned to her face. She could barely keep her eyes open, so we left her with a promise to return first thing in the morning.

For the next two days, physical therapists worked with Mom twice a day to get her to be able to stand and walk, even a few steps. One session would prove promising while the next a complete failure.

I asked for a consultation with a palliative care doctor.

It appeared likely that Mom's inability to bear her own weight was more a function of the brain than the leg muscles. Yes, she was weak, but it seemed clear that, at least sometimes, the legs simply could not receive the brain signal. Even the "Beer Barrel Polka" trick failed.

The doctor's perspective confirmed my intuition as I mentally replayed signs of her decline over the last few months. The increased mental confusion, the loss of appetite, the loss of spark, the difficulty in getting out of her chair, her unsteady steps. I knew. Now I desperately needed him to tell me what to expect next. How did this go? She was obviously failing rapidly, but how long might it last? How did we know when it was time for palliative care?

He did his best to answer my questions, but most answers started with "it depends." His best guess was six months to two years.

After one failed therapy session, Mom and I were alone in her room. She looked at me, sitting at the foot of her bed, and said in her best don't-argue-with-me Mom voice, "I'm done. I'm an old woman. I cannot do this anymore." She repeated, "I'm done."

"Okay, Mom," I replied. "I hear you. You have the right to refuse therapy, and if that's what you want, we will honor it. If that's the case, then we've arrived at the scenario we discussed. If you can't walk, it's time for skilled nursing care."

She nodded.

"Okay, then. I need to talk to the rest of the family, and we'll make a plan."

That evening, the siblings conferred by phone and talked through our options. At first, we thought she would be happier in Casper, Wyoming, where my brothers lived. She would be surrounded by a whole tribe of loving grandchildren. But getting her there would be quite a challenge, and the sudden possibility of assuming responsibility for her care was daunting to my brothers. But Elaine had already cleared her schedule and made arrangements to care for Mom, and that made Indiana look like the best option.

We reviewed the information we had gathered on skilled nursing facilities in each location and made some calls. As it turned out, Joplin was a hot spot for the Delta variant of COVID at that time, and all the local facilities were on lockdown. That ruled out Joplin. Indiana had no lockdowns at the time, and they had availability at Green Valley, a facility less than two miles from my sister's home. We quickly made arrangements to hold a space for her there.

Then it became a matter of transporting her, a nine-hour drive. We knew we would not be able to get her in and out of the car for bathroom stops since she could not stand. She had been catheterized in the hospital, so we decided to leave the catheter in place until we settled her in her new place.

With the assistance of two strong nurses, we managed to get her loaded into the car on the morning of June 22. We stopped by home long enough for Mom to say goodbye to Roger and Rawley. Even though we had explained the plan, her mind didn't fully absorb the magnitude of those goodbyes. In her weakened state, she only knew she was off on a road trip adventure with her girls. She smiled, donned her sunglasses, sat back, and relaxed. She was happy to go anywhere with her girls.

We pulled into the Green Valley parking lot nine hours later, then spent the evening signing paperwork, unloading her belongings, and getting her settled into her room. Exhausted and confused, she took comfort in seeing her quilt on her bed and photos of all her children on the nightstand.

Mom was particularly fond of a small stuffed moose named Cody that Elaine had given her. For years, I had propped him up on her pillow every morning when I made her bed. Cody made the trip to Indiana with her, and we snuggled him next to her when we kissed her goodnight that first night in her new home.

From that day until the day she died nearly six months later, Cody never left her side. Waking or sleeping, Cody was on duty, nestled in the crook of her elbow or sharing her pillow. It killed us to leave her that night, and every night thereafter, but Cody's faithful presence gave us comfort too. Thanks to our fiber-filled proxy, she was never really alone.

I stayed for two days, then flew home just in time to pack and leave for our family trip to Wyoming. Roger and I had planned several trips during the six months we expected Mom to be at Elaine's, and we kept our plans. After long months of COVID isolation, we were desperate for time with our children and grandchildren. Still, it took everything in me to pass the baton to my sister, even though I knew Mom was in good hands. I returned to Indiana between trips, spending at least a week each month, and we did daily FaceTime calls.

Mama was never not on my mind.

13
Green Valley

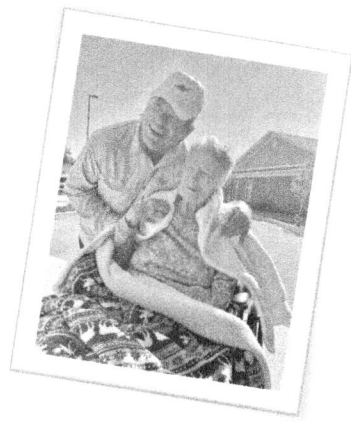

Elaine spent most of each day with Mom, and their lives began to settle into a rhythm. On days when her mind was clear, Mom felt sad and lonely. She begged Elaine, "Can't you take me to your house?"

Elaine explained again that she couldn't care for Mom without help. But she had an idea. Maybe they could bust her out for a short visit on July Fourth. It would be almost like old times, grilling burgers and sipping root beer floats together.

So, they did. Without permission and with no small effort, Dan and Elaine managed to load Mom into their SUV and take her to their house for a visit. I was at the Fourth of July parade in Dubois when I opened a text to see a photo of Mom, sitting in her recliner at Elaine's house, smiling broadly.

Mom didn't have any interest in the burgers, but she could never refuse a root beer float. She sipped away in bliss, and for a moment, all the effort seemed worthwhile. But then Elaine started hearing ominous rumbles from Mom's direction.

It suddenly dawned on her that Mom's stomach, unaccustomed to food, was in no condition to deal with a root beer float. And she hadn't thought to bring any spare clothes. A sudden bout of diarrhea would be disastrous.

In a panic, they cut the visit short and wrangled Mom back into the car. To her dismay, Mom soon found herself back in her bed at Green Valley. None of us liked the separation, but after that adventure, it was very clear Mom was where she needed to be.

From the beginning, the staff at Green Valley loved Mom. She had a whole closet of beautiful clothes and insisted on wearing matching earrings each day.

"You're never really dressed until you have your earrings on," Mom advised Jessica and Margaret, two of her favorite aides.

It became a contest between Jessica and Margaret to see who would get to Mom first each morning and pick out her outfit and earrings. We had our frustrations with the administration at Green Valley, but we came to dearly love the aides and nurses who cared for Mom so well. They were angels of mercy to her and, by extension, to us.

Green Valley did its own assessments of Mom's physical and mental state and decided to try physical therapy again. The ability to stand and walk, even a little, would make her life so much better. I had zero hope that it would help, but given Elaine's enthusiasm, Mom was willing to try.

After two weeks, the physical therapist told us it was time to stop. Mom would occasionally have a good therapy day, but just like our experience at the hospital, the next session would be a complete failure. The trouble, as we suspected, could not be addressed with better muscle tone. Dementia had disrupted the neural pathways from the brain to her legs, and no amount of therapy would change it.

We got the report after I had returned to Indiana from our vacation, so Elaine and I processed it together. It was the answer I had expected, especially after seeing Mom's mobility decline over the last few months, so I was mentally prepared for it. Elaine was not. She wanted so desperately for Mom to get better, and she questioned the decision to give up. In the end, however, the therapist's assessment trumped our opinions. If a patient could not demonstrate steady progress, Medicare would no longer pay for the service. It was out of our hands.

Mom was relieved. She had been willing to try the therapy again but had found it deeply frustrating. In her clearer moments, she would express again that she was "done."

She was also done eating. She refused food at every meal, sometimes swallowing a few bites just to make Elaine happy. The staff brought her protein drinks, and we tried to tempt her with milkshakes and maple bars, but she had no interest in food.

In conversations with Elaine, I reminded her that Mom's disinterest in food began a few months before her fall in June. From my research and my discussion with the palliative care doctor, this was a common occurrence. It was the body's natural course of winding down. Whether Mom's refusal was fully rational or merely instinctual, I believed we should let her call the shots and stop trying to force food into her.

Elaine couldn't get there. It felt like a grievous betrayal to sit by and watch our mother starve herself to death. I was Mom's medical power of attorney, but Elaine oversaw her day-to-day care and needed to be able to follow her own conscience. We settled into a compromise neither of us found wholly satisfactory. When I was there, we backed off on food pressure, but Elaine made her best efforts during the weeks I was absent.

At one point, when Elaine had been trying to coax food into her, she leaned down over Mom's bed for a face-to-face word.

"Mama, you are so skinny," she scolded.

"Oh, honey," Mom whispered. "I've waited all my life to hear those words!"

In the end, it didn't really matter. The small bites of food Mom consumed were not enough calories to sustain her, and she steadily lost weight. Nature had the last word.

It was frustrating that Elaine and I held such divergent positions on the food issue, but I came to understand that her fierce desire to see Mom regain some physical strength was a manifestation of her grief. I was many months ahead of Elaine in my grieving and had already arrived at acceptance. But living with the daily reality of losing Mom was new to Elaine, and her grief was real and raw. In addition, I had been able to make many memories with Mom over the last several years. No wonder Elaine was not ready to let her go. I may not have been either had the roles been reversed.

When Elaine returned to her teaching schedule in August, she keenly felt the pressure of trying to care for Mom and keep up with her classroom. She lived with the tension of never feeling she was giving her best to anyone.

For all the difficulty, however, Elaine loved connecting with the staff and residents at Green Valley. Naturally outgoing, she soon befriended each of the aides and nurses. Many struggled with their own personal pain—a failing marriage, a cancer diagnosis, financial hardship—even as they cared for our mother so tenderly.

Elaine got to know the other residents in Mom's hall, too, whose antics never failed to provide a little levity in that otherwise sad facility. There was Dottie, who got busted for blaring vulgar music one day. And Mary, who always sweetly stalked the halls in her shower cap and one day asked Elaine to help her find her toothbrush. Betty must have been a choir director in her earlier life, Elaine mused, because she serenaded every hallway in the building, singing with gusto all day long.

Barbara made her way across the hall one evening to seek Mom's advice.

"Well, I'm ready to go to bed, but I can't because of all those people in my bed," she said. "Just look at all of them," she gestured toward her room across the hall. "What am I going to do?"

"Well, I would just ask them to scoot over," Mom suggested.

"I never thought of that," Barbara replied. And off she went to bed.

On Sundays, Elaine dressed Mom from head to toe in her Denver Broncos fan wear. On a walk in the courtyard one Sunday afternoon, they encountered Mom's neighbor, Don, similarly garbed in Dallas Cowboy gear. After some mild trash-talking, Elaine suggested a wheelchair race to Don and his daughter, a friendly way to settle the rivalry! I don't recall who won the race, but Elaine reported a lot of laughter and a few squeals of terror from Mom, who never liked to go fast.

Most of the residents were compliant and cooperative, but not all. Two in particular, Evelyn and Jane, protested their loss of autonomy by routinely resisting the establishment.

One afternoon, Elaine's son Nick stopped by to see Mom. A deputy sheriff standing at six feet and eight inches, Nick made an impression when he walked down the hall in his uniform. To his surprise, Evelyn stopped him and began a long explanation, punctuated with frequent assertions that "I didn't do it."

Nick listened patiently, nodded gravely at the appropriate times, and assured her he'd look into it. Then she dropped the bomb.

"Jane has a knife," she said. She went on to explain that Jane had been responsible for the carving in one of the community room tables. "I didn't do it," she asserted again.

Nick passed the information along, not really believing the story, but it turned out to be true! Jane was not happy to lose her knife!

Mom's physical and mental state veered erratically from day to day. One day her mind would be clear and she would express an interest in taking a walk outside or working on a puzzle in the community room. But often, she was in a fog. She slumped in her wheelchair and couldn't wait to be back in her bed.

At first, she required only one aide to transfer her from bed to her chair. She quickly graduated to being a two-person lift, and then shortly thereafter required the mechanical sling lift for transfers. An accident during a two-person lift left her with a long, deep gash on her leg. It took months of intensive wound care to get it to heal.

Elaine had her hands full. Mom constantly fought urinary tract infections and constipation. Before long, she developed nasty bed sores. Her incontinence required frequent changes of clothing and bedding. Elaine took her soiled laundry home each night.

It should have been routine to address each of Mom's medical challenges. After all, we had been assured that a team of three doctors and a physician's assistant oversaw the medical needs of the residents, and a registered nurse was always on duty. Their photos and credentials had been featured prominently in the glossy Green Valley brochure.

As it turned out, communication and processes were poor. The nurse on duty often had no notes from the prior shift. Resident files were kept in large three-ring binders with no digital records. It might be three days before lab results were filed into the notebook, and no one could access them until the filing got caught up. It was enormously frustrating.

For all the hours we spent present with Mom over nearly six months, we saw a doctor only one time. He stood in the doorway, gave me a quick update on wound care for one of her bed sores, and then scurried away. The whole exchange took less than two minutes. As much time as we spent in the building, it was curious that we never even accidentally crossed paths with one of the three doctors. Maybe they made rounds in the middle of the night? Or did they make them at all?

Elaine occasionally saw the physician's assistant, who assured her that a doctor was monitoring Mom's bed sores and her leg wound. But details were elusive. We asked for an itemized list of the charges that were billed to Medicare monthly. Then after a few days, we asked again. When we finally held the invoice in our hands, sure enough, there were numerous charges for doctor visits.

Elaine followed up to request the notes from those doctor visits. And then she followed up again. We never received the notes.

In July, Elaine recognized that Mom had a urinary tract infection. It took five days to get a lab confirmation, and by that time, Mom was out of her head and Elaine was out of patience. She insisted that Mom be given IV antibiotics immediately.

With fluids and antibiotics, Mom perked up and became her old self again. Just in time, because all four siblings and a dear friend from Colorado had gathered in Indiana to see her that weekend. We celebrated my brother Steve's birthday, and Mom even tried to enjoy a bite or two of his German chocolate cake. Surrounded by so many of her loves, Mom rallied and had several days of mental clarity before slipping back into a fog.

I could sense her confusion one morning as she asked me questions. Not only was she unsure who we were sometimes, but she wasn't entirely clear on who *she* was. I picked up a framed photo on her nightstand and handed it to her. It was the "glamor shot" photo we had done with Mitzi four years earlier. Looking back at her from the frame were three laughing women, beautifully dressed and carefree. She raised her eyes to look at me and, pointing to her image in the photo, said in amazement, "That's me! That's me and my girls!"

"Yes, Mama. That's you! That's us," I said through tears. "If you're ever having trouble remembering who you are, just look at that photo and you'll remember how much fun we had that day."

She smiled and settled into her pillows.

I usually brought Rawley with me on trips to see Mom. We created a happy stir among the residents every time we came and went, and I wondered if Rawley might have a promising future as a therapy dog. A comfort coonhound... Yes, I could see it! She certainly was good for Mom. At each visit, Rawley would jump up on Mom's bed and kiss her face to shrieks of delight, then stretch her long body out next to Mom's and settle in for a nap.

When I came in September, I brought Mom another stuffed moose. Roger and I had just returned from a trip to Sheridan, Wyoming, a place that held many memories for us all. We named the moose Sheridan, and he became Cody's playmate. Sometimes we'd step into the room to find Mom talking earnestly to Cody and Sheridan. After I left, Mom confessed to Elaine that she thought Sheridan was a little "funny-looking." She welcomed him more for Cody's benefit than her own, she explained. Cody would always be her favorite.

I never knew what to expect on my visits to see Mom. She was always excited to see me, but in September she couldn't recall my name. She lit up when I came through the door and told the aide, "That's my mother! She took me into her home and took care of me!"

By the end of September, it was clear that Mom's quality of life had deteriorated dramatically. She loved seeing us, but she spent most of her hours alone in spite of our best efforts. On mentally clear days, even Cody could not reassure her. Dementia provided a sweet relief from her loneliness.

When I walked into her room on one of her clear mornings, she implored with the saddest face, "When are we going home?"

Home was always Joplin. Our house. And she might not be able to recall my name, but she never forgot the feeling of safety and belonging she had experienced in our home. She longed to go back to those days.

Given the rare opportunity of her mental clarity, I broached the topic on our minds.

"Mama," I began tentatively, "I know you desperately want me to take you home to Joplin, but I think the day may be coming soon when you get to go Home, to your ultimate home. With Jesus."

Her eyes widened in surprise, and she said, "Am I that bad?"

"Well, you're not getting better, Mama. You don't want to eat, and that's fine, but you're getting weaker every day. I think your body is winding down, and I don't know anything that's going to turn it around. So, while you're having a pretty good day today, I think overall, you're not getting better."

She thought for just a second, absorbing that news, and then said, "Well, then I say 'Hallelujah!'"

We laughed together and she said, "I'm going to get to see my mother. And Jesus."

"Yes, Mama, you are," I said through tears. "It will be a happy day for you. When you get your new body, your legs will be strong again, your mind will be clear, and you'll be happy. We're going to miss you like crazy when you go Home, but some sweet day we'll all be together again."

I remembered one of our conversations from a few weeks earlier. She knew how much it bothered me that I couldn't be with her all the time, and I think she had been trying to comfort me.

"You know, He talks to me," she had said.

"Who, Mama? Jesus?"

"Yes. We talk," she had replied. "He tells me everything is going to be all right. He's always with me."

During one of her hallucinations earlier, she had also told me the clock on the wall talked to her, but I knew this one was different. Her mind was clear that day, and her countenance peaceful. It didn't surprise me a lick that Jesus had been talking to her. Of course He had. They were tight.

Knowing Mom's outlook on her final days gave us comfort, but we were still troubled. Where did we go from here, we wondered. Was it time to pursue palliative care? Hospice? We spoke to the Green Valley director, and she cheerfully scheduled a meeting with herself, the director of nursing, and two other staff members who could advise us and answer our questions. On the day of the meeting, none of them showed up. A nurse's aide finally came in late, made some half-hearted apologies, and did her best to address our questions. Clearly, we would have to figure it out ourselves.

I would have opted for hospice at that point, but Elaine had seen the hospice representative coming and going at the facility—a twenty-something with pink hair. She emphatically expressed a hard pass on the hospice option.

Ultimately, we settled on palliative care and advised the nursing director of our decision. We were not entirely certain how our decision would play out, but we expressed our intention to take Mom off almost all her medications and focus on comfort and pain relief. We stopped her Warfarin (blood thinner), which gave her relief from twice weekly blood draws that had become torturous. We still wanted to treat her urinary tract infections, for the sake of her comfort. She was drinking very little, but we opted against any IV fluids. Her nurses assured us that, when the time came, we would be able to approve the use of narcotics to ease any suffering.

I thought of the Dylan Thomas poem, "Do Not Go Gentle into That Good Night," which begins:

> *Do not go gentle into that good night,*
> *Old age should burn and rave at close of day;*
> *Rage, rage against the dying of the light.*

Suddenly, I saw the poem for what it is, the anguished cry of a son desperate not to lose his father. I could see Dylan Thomas shoveling applesauce between his dad's parched lips, coaxing him to accept sustenance. I could see him begging some faceless power not to give up on physical therapy. Dylan Thomas was us. But now we had turned a corner. Now we vowed to walk with Mama—gently, oh gently we prayed—into that good night.

Aside from changes to her medication, life continued much the same after our decision. Mostly, we had settled in our own minds that we were ready to let nature take its course. Loving her well meant letting her go. We had not arrived at the decision quickly, and we had honored Mom's agency as best we could. Even so, our hearts were heavy. I found reassurance in the fact that we had arrived at the decision together.

Months before, I had booked our favorite cabin in Dubois for nearly three weeks in October. I was torn, but Roger and I decided to keep our plans, expecting to cut them short if Mom began to fail quickly. Now, more than ever, I needed to step away from the world for a space.

As I kissed her goodbye, I promised to be back soon. My heart hurt, but I knew she was in good hands.

14
Once More to the Wild

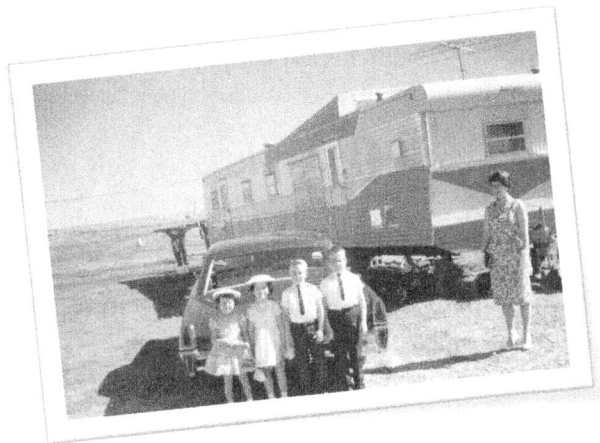

AS SOON AS WE HAD settled on the six-month caregiving rotation with Elaine, I started longing for a soul retreat. Eighteen months of pandemic isolation, Mom's failing health, and the loss of a close friendship had left me thoroughly depleted. I needed time alone, in nature. Time to rest and read and pray and nap. Time when no one needed anything from me.

Roger understood. I booked our Dubois cabin for seventeen days in late October. We planned for me to spend the first twelve days by myself, and then he would fly to Jackson and join me for the last five days. We would drive home together.

As the date drew near, I invited two girlfriends to join me for three days in the middle of my solitude. I wasn't sure I could handle that much of my own company, and I knew they would be good for my soul. They were.

I packed warm clothes, my camera, a cooler of frozen soup, homemade granola, and a pile of books. Simplicity ruled. Then Rawley and I pulled out of the driveway for our eighteen-hour solo trip. We arrived the next afternoon and unpacked the weight of the world.

The little ranching community of Dubois has been a bright thread woven through our family for more than forty years. Without a single traffic light or fast-food restaurant, Dubois invites its guests to relax. Exhale. Breathe deeply the sage-scented air.

The simplicity of the town echoes its residents. Unpretentious, grounded folks. Friendly without being in your business. Rolling through town, I returned the two-fingered wave of every passing pickup. This enduring symbol of Western neighborliness sure took me back. I was home.

I stopped at the Super Foods IGA, the only grocery store in town, to pick up milk and bread and eggs. Main Street was quiet. Most visitors at this time of year wore camouflage and orange vests. Our two favorite restaurants were closed for two weeks while their owners went hunting for elk and deer. Good thing I had brought my soup.

With my comfort coonhound at my side, our days settled into a rhythm. Rise with the sun, linger over coffee, read. Take a walk down the gravel road to the Wind River, chatting with the neighbor horses on the way. After a soup lunch, go for a drive, camera in hand, on the lookout for wildlife and adventure. Come home, take a nap, work on a puzzle, and warm up another bowl of soup for supper.

It was my first time to be in Dubois so late in the year, and I was afraid the fall color would be gone. But no! Vibrant golds tangled with bare silvery branches to create a mysterious landscape. On our glorious walks and drives, I let the peace sink deep into my bones.

But all that thinking time led to some less-than-peaceful introspection too. Everyone knows the first rule of caregiving is self-care. And on the off chance I had somehow missed Rule Number One, well-meaning friends and family had often reminded me. So, how had I let myself get into this state?

Certainly, the pandemic had played a large role, especially since it had coincided with Mom's accelerated decline. Sheer fatigue played a role as well. It wasn't like I didn't know I needed to care for my own well-being; I simply couldn't muster the energy. After a while, I had chafed at the well-intended reminders about self-care.

But I had to admit that my own sense of duty and invincibility also played a role. I was strong. I was fine. Really. There's a reason firstborn daughters often default to the caregiving role. We're responsible from the day we're born. And sometimes we have control issues.

With new perspective, I saw the last year of my life as a Chinese finger trap. We had played with these braided bamboo cylinders as children, urging each other to stick a finger into the cylinder and then pull it back out. Once in, however, any effort to pull your finger out causes the cylinder to tighten. The only way out is to push your finger forward, counterintuitively, which causes the braid to relax. Then you can squeeze the cylinder together and easily remove your finger.

I'd been pulling for so long, I couldn't let go. Even now, it was hard to enjoy the quiet relief and let someone else take over Mom's care.

One morning, huge fluffy snowflakes began to fall as I sipped my morning coffee. Without so much as a breeze, each flake twirled pirouettes in graceful descent. Faster and faster they came until I could hardly see the river just a hundred yards from my picture window. Rawley and I applauded the show from our front-row seat on the couch.

The planner in me suggested this would be a good time to work on Mom's obituary while I had time to think and reflect. I flipped through photos, some on my laptop and some in my memory, trying to find words to capture the lovely woman I called Mama.

I thought about her courage and resilience. As a young widow with two small boys, she had known deep sorrow. After marrying my dad, she had quickly added two little girls to the mix. My dad's job in the oilfield had taken him out of town for long stretches and had required us to pull up stakes and move our trailer house many times. Virtually a single parent for much of our childhood, she had nonetheless made our home-on-wheels a happy place.

One photo in particular captured her essence and our childhood perfectly. Taken on Easter morning, the photo revealed the four of us dressed in our finery, standing in front of our 1965 Mercury Marquis before heading to church. Our green Artcraft trailer house in the background didn't have any skirting, so you could see the blocks propping it up underneath. The yard was just bare dirt, not a tree, shrub, or plant anywhere in sight. It could have been any one of the many windswept Wyoming oil towns we had called home. Behind the trailer, a single pair of my dad's coveralls hung on the clothesline.

Never mind the bleak background, Elaine and I proudly sported ruffled dresses, white anklet socks, patent Mary Janes, and little purses. Our hair fell in tight ringlets beneath white straw hats, the result of sleeping in pink foam rollers. Steve and Andy stood at attention in dark slacks, white shirts, and clip-on striped ties, their close-cropped hair slicked back to perfection. Their shoes were shined. And off to the side, barely in the photo, was Mama. She was all beauty and grace in a flower-print sheath dress, heels, pearls, and white gloves, her Bible tucked under one arm. And the look on her face? She simply adored us.

Mama was a woman who knew Jesus as a friend, not an abstraction. I remembered peeking my small head around her bedroom door many times, only to find her kneeling by her bed in prayer. And I can still picture the cover of *Our Daily Bread*, the Bible devotional we read from every morning after breakfast.

For all her Baptist piety, however, the woman loved to dance. She and Daddy had met at a dance, as was common in their day. I smiled to think that perhaps God, because He must have a sense of humor, would see fit to welcome her into glory with a rousing rendition of the "Beer Barrel Polka!" Ironically, dancing was a pastime she denied her children when we became teenagers.

One evening, a few years earlier, Mom and I had been watching *The Lawrence Welk Show* together. As Bobby and Sissy whirled and twirled around the dance floor, she had sighed and said wistfully, "Did you dance when you were young?"

"Seriously?" I replied. "Did I dance? Um… no! I had a good Baptist mama who believed girls who went to dances came home pregnant! So no, I never danced!"

"Oh, that's too bad," she had sympathized, apparently failing to make the connection.

Snuggled with Rawley that snowy day, I replayed memories for hours, but not a single word made it to the page. Words would never do her justice.

Finally, I let go of any expectation to be productive and resigned myself to just being. Hard times lay ahead, but for a few more days, I could allow myself to be suspended in grace.

On the drive to Jackson a few days later, over Togwotee Pass, I saw a grizzly and her two cubs. I knew immediately it was the grizzly known to locals as Felicia. What a thrill to be the only one watching her for several minutes, and so close! On the way home, I stopped to admire a cow moose and calf. Later that week, a black bear jaunted through my yard while I watched him from the window. God knew my deep appreciation for his creatures, and I received each sighting with gratitude.

After Roger joined me, we spent a day exploring back roads in the Tetons, then another day driving through Yellowstone. We were thrilled by the sight of more grizzlies, elk, bison, and moose. It was good to be together.

During those sacred days, I spread the ashes of my grief across the wild places I loved so much, raising both hands open to a faithful God who restores my soul.

15
Going Home

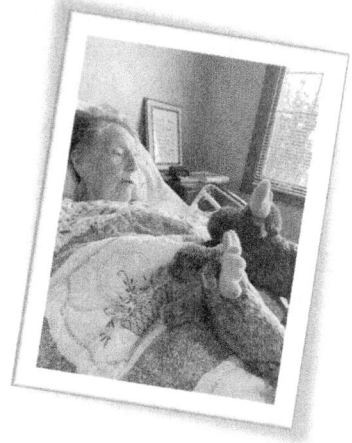

I HAD PLANNED TO RETURN to Indiana in early November, but plans changed. Mom contracted COVID. They had moved her to an insolation wing, and Elaine had to don full hazmat gear every time she went in to see her. No way they would let me in.

Elaine reported that Mom's COVID symptoms were mild, with one exception. She had explosive diarrhea. The difficulty of keeping her clean compounded the seriousness of her bedsores. They had been trying for weeks to grow new skin on one particular sore on her backside, but they could not clean her up several times a day without disrupting the new skin growth. The bedsore was Elaine's gravest concern.

Mom was thin and frail, but had lucid moments and was in decent spirits. I could still FaceTime with her, and Elaine kept me updated on her interactions with the nursing staff. I wanted to be there so badly.

By the time she was released from isolation, it was nearly Thanksgiving and we were preparing our usual large family celebration. After the pandemic had canceled our Thanksgiving gathering the year before, we were anxious to resume one of our favorite traditions.

Mom declined steadily during Thanksgiving week. How long could a body last without food and water, we wondered. Longer than we thought possible. The sore on her backside got worse by the day.

The last of our kids and grandkids left to return home the Saturday after Thanksgiving, November 27. No sooner had I hugged and kissed the last one than I threw my suitcase in the trunk and hit the road for Indiana.

Mama was weak but greeted me with a sweet smile. "Oh, I am so happy to see you."

Elaine and I stayed by her side most of the weekend. Sunday afternoon, we turned the television on to whatever NFL game was playing that day. Normally, Mom was an avid football fan, and we hoped it might provide some distraction for her. Not so. Before long, she said irritably, "For the life of me, I am so sick of watching grown men crash into each other! What is the point of all that?"

Elaine and I laughed and turned the TV off. Out in the hall, we agreed that Mama was ready to see Jesus when she couldn't enjoy a football game!

We desperately needed that moment of levity because the bedsore had become necrotic. The first time I saw it, I thought I might throw up. Mama had a deep hole, the size of a golf ball, on her backside. The skin all around it had turned black and smelled like roadkill. God bless nurses.

Mama slept most of the time, clutching Cody tight. On Tuesday, one of the nurses came in to tend to her. The nurse leaned down close to Mama's ear, and said, "Norma, we're going to turn you over, sweetie."

She opened her eyes and whispered, "Please don't hurt me."

"That's it," I told Elaine in the hall. "It's time to start the morphine. She's clearly in pain, and I cannot watch her suffer."

We started a morphine dosing schedule that night, and Elaine and I look back on that decision with one big regret. We didn't have a conversation with Mom, one final chance to tell her how much we loved her before we started the morphine. She was so rarely lucid and awake by that time that our only thought was to start the morphine quickly to ease her suffering.

We kept our friends and family apprised with occasional Facebook posts. On December first, I wrote:

> These are tender days. I woke up sobbing at 4 a.m., dread plopping its bulky mass in the middle of my chest. Elaine had a similar night. Coffee in hand, we head into the dark, making our way to Mama. Elaine needs to lay eyes on her before she heads to school.
>
> Two hours later, my Fitbit nags me: it's time to move. But I am rooted in this chair, watching the raggedy rise and fall of Mama's bony chest. Yesterday she opened her eyes, smiled, and whispered, "I am so glad to see you." But yesterday was pre-morphine, and that may have been our last sunburst through these clouds.
>
> Acoustic Christmas music softly competes with the noise in the hall. I massage a silky aromatherapy cream into Mama's parched arms, smear Vaseline on her cracked lips, stroke her hair, and tell her she's the best mom in the world.
>
> Two days ago, she accepted a few bites of my homemade applesauce. It took us back to sun-dappled Colorado days when the apple trees in her back yard nearly broke beneath the weight of their harvest. We are beyond applesauce today.
>
> 'I read the Psalms to her, especially Psalm 23. She gives no outward response, but I know the words are soul aromatherapy, soaking deep below the conscious mind. I'm confident she can see the table set before her, and she yearns to dwell in the house of the Lord forever. Home. Soon.
>
> Emmanuel, God with us. Yes, these are tender days.

We couldn't leave her now. Elaine got a substitute to cover her classes, and we took shifts sitting with her. We were midwives, birthing our Mama into her next life. Full circle. We come into the world through pain and travail, and we leave in much the same way. At least she was no longer suffering.

We quietly discussed our next steps. Mom would be cremated, and we would bury her next to Daddy in Longmont, Colorado. We started looking at dates and contacting the funeral home and family members to float various possibilities. We talked about the service and how we could best honor her. We wanted everyone to have a chance to participate if they wanted to. Elaine's husband, Dan, was a minister, and he agreed to do the service.

We wanted to do something for the Green Valley staff who cared for Mom so lovingly. Elaine had spent so much time there over the past six months that she had grown close to several of the aides and nurses. One day, she found the perfect keepsake on an Etsy website—a Christmas ornament made from a slice of tree branch with a moose and birch trees wood-burned into the surface. Perfect! We counted how many we would need to give one to each of the Green Valley staff and to every guest we expected at her service, then contacted the artisan to see if they could make such a large quantity on short notice. They were happy to help.

For four days, we sat with Mama. We didn't suppose she could hear us, but we talked to her and played the acoustic Christmas CD she loved so much. We rubbed lotion on her thin arms and held her hand. Elaine wrote thank-you notes to each of the staff members during our vigil. We had moments of shared reminiscing, but I mostly recall it as a quiet, heavy time. Yes, we tended to details we knew would demand our attention soon, but it felt almost profane to turn our attention too long from the task at hand.

Late in the evening on December 4, Mama took a deep breath, let it go with a strong exhale, and walked through the veil. Safely home.

16
A Love Remembered

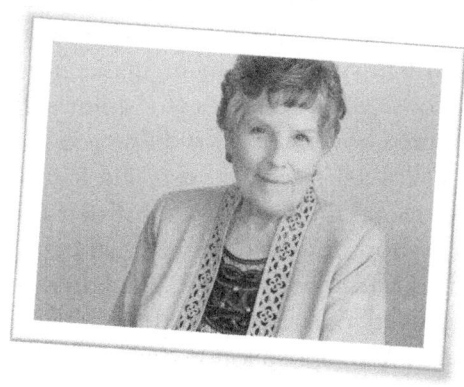

I SHOULD HAVE FELT RELIEVED. And I did, at some level. We had passed through the "valley of the shadow of death" and emerged on the other side. No longer would that looming anxiety dog my every step and rob me of my sleep. Mama had been liberated from her broken body and was now safely beyond the reach of pain. *Yes*, I told myself, *that's a relief.*

But my heart could not get on the same page. Mama had gone Home, but she had been my home all my life. Now she was gone, leaving me orphaned and homeless. Would I ever feel anchored and safe and loved completely again? I desperately needed to crawl into her lap and feel her gently stroke my hair. Only she could make me believe everything would be okay.

After days of helpless inactivity, at least now we had something to do. My inner planner leaped into action. I went home, and Elaine worked with the local funeral home to get the official death certificate and arrange cremation. I finally found words for her obituary, secured the funeral home in Colorado for her service, made hotel and plane reservations, and contacted friends.

Mom had left us no instructions for her service. Her one request, we learned, came through her dear friend, Mary Lou. Mom loved drums, and Mary Lou's son, Jimmy, sometimes played the drums during worship at her church. Mom adored Jimmy and had told Mary Lou she wanted him to play the drums at her funeral.

As uncommon as drum solos at funerals might be, we would honor her request. We selected For King and Country's rendition of "The Little Drummer Boy," appropriate for the Christmas season. Jimmy played it with a gusto so atypical for funeral music that we still laugh at the memory. Mom would have loved it.

Some of Mom's granddaughters wanted to participate in the service. Hannah, a gifted pianist, offered a solo; Cierra and Gracie wanted to share funny memories; and Leah would read Psalm 23. Elaine and I both wanted to speak. Dan prepared the eulogy. Roger didn't want to speak, but my remarks included a tribute to him. He had gone above and beyond in his loving care for Mom.

In another departure from convention, we decided to serve root beer floats, her favorite treat, at the reception afterward. The moose ornaments, our keepsake gift for the guests, arrived just in time. Piece by piece, the service came together.

The final item on the program would be a photo slideshow, leaving us with a montage of memories. My siblings searched their albums and computers and sent me their favorite photos while I searched for the music. It had to be just right.

I couldn't find what I wanted and was nearing panic when I finally happened upon Steffany Gretzinger's version of "No One Ever Cared for Me Like Jesus." It was perfect.

On the day of her service, I looked out over the sea of faces.

The neighbor who had given her a box of See's chocolates every Christmas and Easter since her stroke in 2008.

Another neighbor who had mowed her lawn and tended the garden after Daddy died.

Her friends from the antiques business who had saved front-row seats for her at every auction.

Her dear Sunday School class ladies with whom she had laughed and cried for many years.

Her financial advisor and his assistant who had become like family.

Grown-up "kids" who had passed their teenage years playing ping pong and poker in her basement.

They had all found love and acceptance when their lives had intersected with hers. In turn, she was so loved.

As the service neared its close, I turned our guests' attention to the screen.

"Mama's faith was so deeply embedded into her heart and mind, even dementia couldn't touch it," I said. "She didn't always know *who* she was, but she always knew *whose* she was. She's here with us today, in spirit, and her parting message to us is in this song, so listen closely."

The lyrics spoke of the never-ending love of God, how that was the anchoring joy of her life, and how it was the legacy she wished to pass on to her children and grandchildren. It was as if Mom were singing the words herself.

The service ran a little long, but no one cared. With so much love to remember, our guests lingered over their charcuterie board appetizers and root beer floats. We celebrated her life, but oh, how we grieved her loss. With both hands open, we honored her.

After all the guests had gone and the final details wrapped up, I stepped outside and looked up into a sky so blue I could hear Mama's voice in my head declaring it "Wyoming blue."

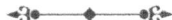

The family had planned an extra day to spend together after the service. We drove up to Estes Park, one of Mom's favorite places, and spent time in quiet conversation. We thought back through every decision on our journey. Had we done the right thing? We couldn't say with certainty. Would we have done anything differently? Yes, some things, to be sure.

As Mom's days approached the end, I had regretted not starting the morphine earlier, but Elaine felt guilty that we had started it when we did. Every decision held an opportunity for guilt or at least self-doubt.

Over the next many months, we would continue to replay every decision. I desperately wished I could have stayed by Mom's side continuously until the end. Should we have tried harder to find a way to keep her at home, maybe with hospice help? I relived every tearful goodbye during the six months she was at Green Valley. Those goodbyes gutted me.

Eventually, I came to see that final transition to Green Valley in a more positive light. It had been brutal for all of us, but it had given Elaine six months of close interaction with Mom she otherwise would not have had. She had reordered her life at no small effort, but I know she would gladly make that sacrifice all over again.

So many things on this journey had not gone the way I had anticipated. Losing my job was traumatic, but it turned out to be a huge relief. Likewise, having to pass the baton to Elaine and missing so much time with Mama in those final months had not been in my plan. And yet, it had given Elaine precious time with Mom. The hard times, viewed from some distance, proved to be grace upon grace.

We all had some healing to do. Roger and I had to get to know one another again and adjust to being a couple. My identity had been "caregiver" for so long that I had to rediscover myself and my purpose. Elaine paid the price in her physical health and spent months recovering from a bacterial infection she contracted from doing Mom's soiled laundry.

These days, Roger and I find ourselves laughing easily. We recently celebrated our forty-fifth wedding anniversary, and I surprised him with a stack of letters he had written to me during our long-distance engagement. He had no idea I had saved them. We spent a couple of hours reading through them that night, remembering small details of our courtship we had long forgotten. It was good to be reminded that, at our core, we were still the same people who had fallen in love so long ago. When our fresh-faced selves had pledged to grow old together, we had no idea. But here we are. Old, and still together. There's a tenderness beneath the battle scars, a compassion for our broken places, and a deep contentment in just being together.

Elaine and I talk frequently and see each other as often as possible. I had secretly worried that we siblings would lose touch with each other without Mama since she was the sun around which we all revolved. Instead, we all find ourselves planning trips, going to great lengths to spend time together. The bond of shared memories has never been stronger. We laugh at every retelling of our childhood stories, but we're also quick to tears. Loss has made us tender souls. Like old people whose paper-thin skin provides scant protection for the body's flesh and sinew, our emotions lie unprotected, close to the surface.

In the end, we came through our caregiving journey with cherished relationships intact. We walked Mama home together. Whatever mistakes we may have made, we find comfort in knowing Mama felt safe and loved in our care. Her years in our home were among the happiest of her life.

I miss her every single day, but here I stand, lifting open hands to receive both grief and joy with a grateful heart.

Afterward

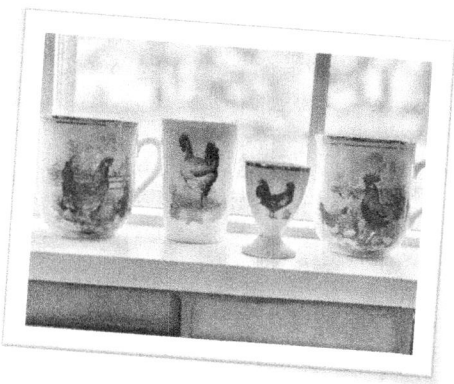

I NEVER LIKED CHICKENS. I do, however, have fond memories of waking up to crowing roosters at my grandparents' house in Sheridan, Wyoming. Grandpa had many roosters, all in separate wire-framed pens. They strutted around their confines, parading brilliant iridescent plumes. Proud, even in confinement. Defiant. Throwing back their delicate combed heads, opening wide their orange beaks, and belting out a challenge to the sun, long before its rising.

Even now, fifty years later, people remember Grandpa's chickens. I stopped by the old place with two cousins to reminisce last summer. The current owner agreed to let us walk around the yard and relive our memories. Though she had never met my grandfather, she immediately recalled with a raised eyebrow, "Ah, yes, he was the one with the roosters." Yes. Also known as fighting cocks. A gruesome sport, cock fighting was every bit as illegal then as it is today, and that's why people remember Grandpa fifty years later. All I remember were the large trophies and pre-dawn crowing.

Grandpa had nicer chickens too. Hens. Basket in hand, we kids had been dispatched to the coop to gather eggs on summer mornings. Funny thing about hens—they really aren't that nice. Turns out they don't relinquish their precious eggs without a great deal of squawking and flapping and fluttering. To my everlasting relief, my egg-gathering days had ended when Grandpa stepped out of the coop one morning with a writhing black snake plucked from its hiding place in the straw. From that day forward, we could all pretend I was afraid of snakes, not chickens.

Mama, on the other hand, loved chickens. She grew up to pre-dawn rooster crows, and thus she never met a rooster who didn't remind her of the father she adored. Her Colorado kitchen had been a veritable chicken shrine, every surface and corner displaying her collection of feathered friends. The set of fine china cups with hand-painted roosters and hens was her favorite.

The rooster cup collection survived the downsizing to her apartment in Missouri, and then a year later they found a home on my kitchen windowsill when she moved in with us. How many times had she steered her walker around the kitchen island, doing laps, and stopping when she passed the rooster cups? I lost count.

"Oh, my rooster cups!" she'd exclaim. "I remember these! They remind me of my daddy."

It's been two years since we walked Mama home.

I reclaimed our bedroom, painting it a calming sage green and replacing Mama's Victorian decor with mementos that evoke my love for nature. We distributed her last remaining possessions within the family, but I was not ready to part with the rooster cups. I may never be ready. I find myself stopping often in front of that windowsill, remembering the mother I adored.

I picture my own children someday, after my funeral, facing those cups on the windowsill. "Who wants the chickens?" they'll ask. They don't think they like chickens right now but just wait. Grief is a trickster, and they may discover an odd affection for chickens after all. I did.

Acknowledgments

Without the encouragement and contributions of many people, this book would have remained in my head. I'm grateful for every encouraging word and every thoughtful critique that shaped the development of our story.

Special thanks to Jonathan Rogers, who played the unenviable role of developmental editor. He saw the roughest of rough drafts and knew exactly where to challenge me. Without his constructive feedback at that early stage, this book would have been a far lesser offering.

I'm grateful for a dreamy week on the Wind River Indian Reservation in Wyoming that led to my friendship with Karen Gilliland and Margaret Coel. A skilled editor, Karen helped me further develop and polish my second draft. Margaret, a *New York Times* bestselling author and my fangirl crush, generously made time to read the manuscript and endorse it. Karen and Margaret's enthusiasm for the book spurred me on when I started to doubt its value. I'm deeply grateful for their generosity.

What fabulous good luck led me to find Kara Wilson at Emerging Ink Solutions? Possibly the world's best copyeditor, not much gets past her eagle eye. Her idea for the cover design was brilliant, and she patiently walked me through every step of the publishing process. It was a delight to collaborate with someone so skilled, so professional, and so kind.

Many thanks to Leslie Roberts, that rare friend who volunteers to read an early draft. She is one of the few people I would ever let see such a rough work in progress! Her encouragement and constructive feedback came at just the right time.

I owe a debt of gratitude to Toni Cutbirth, Barb Owsley, and Stephanie Bracken, who loved my mama and gave me critical respite time. Their friendship brightened her world, as well as mine. Likewise, Dr. Stephen Thomas and the staff at Green Valley were angels of mercy to us.

Of course, I'm especially thankful for my siblings, Steve Bartosh, Andy Bartosh, and Elaine Smith. From earliest childhood, I've always been able to count on their support. We may never agree on who started the Great Schulenburg Tomato War, but all is forgiven.

Most of all, I'm grateful for my husband, Roger. Very few men would have cared for their mother-in-law so tenderly. His wisdom, generosity of spirit, and good humor carried us. I'm blessed to have him by my side.

Lastly, I treasure the many friends who walked this journey with us. Too many to name individually, their friendship and encouragement mean the world to me.

About the Author

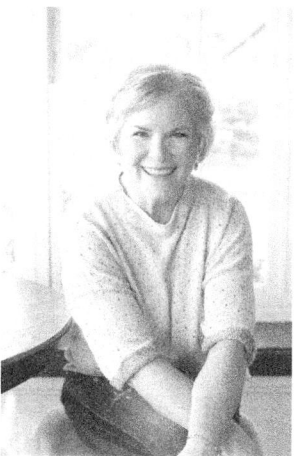

From the time she read her first chapter book, Aileen has loved language and story. She dreamed of college and writing but deferred those dreams to marry her sweetheart at age eighteen. Together, they left their beloved Wyoming roots and ministered at a children's home in Oklahoma for fourteen years, adding three children to their family along the way.

In her thirties, Aileen finally pursued her college education, graduating with degrees in English and Communication just as her firstborn graduated high school. Once again, she postponed her writing dreams in favor of a more economically viable career in business.

In 2015, her life was upended in the span of six weeks when she lost her father and career and became her mother's caregiver. Ill-prepared for such a role, she spent the next six years learning the art of caregiving and making tender memories with her mother. Their journey took another detour when the confluence of COVID-19 and dementia swept them into deep water.

Aileen describes walking parents through their final years as a "terrifying blessing" and wants to reassure other caregivers that they are not alone on their own unique journeys.

With her mama safely home, Aileen now embraces the dream so long delayed—writing about faith, family, and her love of wild places.

She loves to connect with her readers via her blog at comeonaileenblog.com.

Made in the USA
Monee, IL
21 August 2024

63683909R10073